MAY 1 6 2013

6/17-94

EAST MEADOW PUBLIC LIBRARY

3 1299 00886 4242

W9-DFC-278

7 WEEKS TO 10 POUNDS OF MUSCLE

BRETT STEWART & JASON WARNER

East Meadow Public Library
1886 Front Street, East Meadow, NY 11554
(516) 794-2570
www.eastmeadow.info

THE COMPLETE DAY-BY-DAY PROGRAM TO PACK ON LEAN, HEALTHY MUSCLE MASS

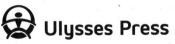 Ulysses Press

To each of our sons, Ian and Luke: True strength comes from compassion, honesty and integrity...but a set of big biceps never hurt either.

Text Copyright © 2013 Brett Stewart and Jason Warner. Design and concept © 2013 Ulysses Press and its licensors. Photographs copyright © 2013 Scott E. Whitney except as noted below. All rights reserved. No part of this publication may be reproduced, stored in a retrieval system, or transmitted in any form or by any means without the prior written permission of the publisher, nor be otherwise circulated in any form of binding or cover other than that in which it is published and without a similar condition being imposed on the subsequent purchaser.

Published in the United States by
ULYSSES PRESS
P.O. Box 3440
Berkeley, CA 94703
www.ulyssespress.com

ISBN13: 978-1-61243-122-2
Library of Congress Control Number 2012951885

Printed in the United States by Bang Printing

10 9 8 7 6 5 4 3 2 1

Contributing Writer: Corey Irwin
Acquisitions Editor: Keith Riegert
Managing Editor: Claire Chun
Editors: Lauren Harrison, Lily Chou
Index: Sayre Van Young
Cover design: what!design @ whatweb.com
Interior photographs: see page 159
Front cover photograph: © Miroslav Georgijevic/istockphoto.com
Back cover photograph: © Anetta/shutterstock.com
Models: Evan Klontz, Brad Mollen, Brett Stewart

Please Note

This book has been written and published strictly for informational purposes, and in no way should be used as a substitute for consultation with health care professionals. You should not consider educational material herein to be the practice of medicine or to replace consultation with a physician or other medical practitioner. The authors and publisher are providing you with information in this work so that you can have the knowledge and can choose, at your own risk, to act on that knowledge. The authors and publisher also urge all readers to be aware of their health status and to consult health care professionals before beginning any health program. This book is independently authored and published and no sponsorship or endorsement of this book by, and no affiliation with, any trademarked events, brands or other products mentioned or pictured within is claimed or suggested. All trademarks that appear in this book belong to their respective owners and are used here for informational purposes only. The authors and publisher encourage readers to patronize the quality events, brands and other products mentioned and pictured in this book.

Table of Contents

Foreword

This book is the culmination of many years of trials, tribulations, research, missteps, exploration and experimentation. The ideas presented are an amalgamation of decades-old knowledge, cutting-edge research, professional industry expertise and our own conclusions based on our results. Throughout you will find overlap with other programs, inspiration from other nutrition regimes, and homage to some of the old-school truths of bodybuilding. We hope you enjoy the ride!

We want to give credit where credit is due. Our workout draws inspiration from many other programs, including Jim Wendler's 5/3/1 (www.jimwendler.com), Dante Trudel's Doggcrapp Training (seriously, that's the name—dc-training.blogspot.com) and the venerable old-school favorite, German Volume Training (GVT).

Our nutrition regime could not have been created without research and exploration done by Martin Berkhan (www.leangains.com), Jason Ferruggia (jasonferruggia .com) and John Kiefer (www.dangerouslyhardcore.com).

A hearty thank you to all of the above for giving to the greater good, which allowed us to create our own humble contribution.

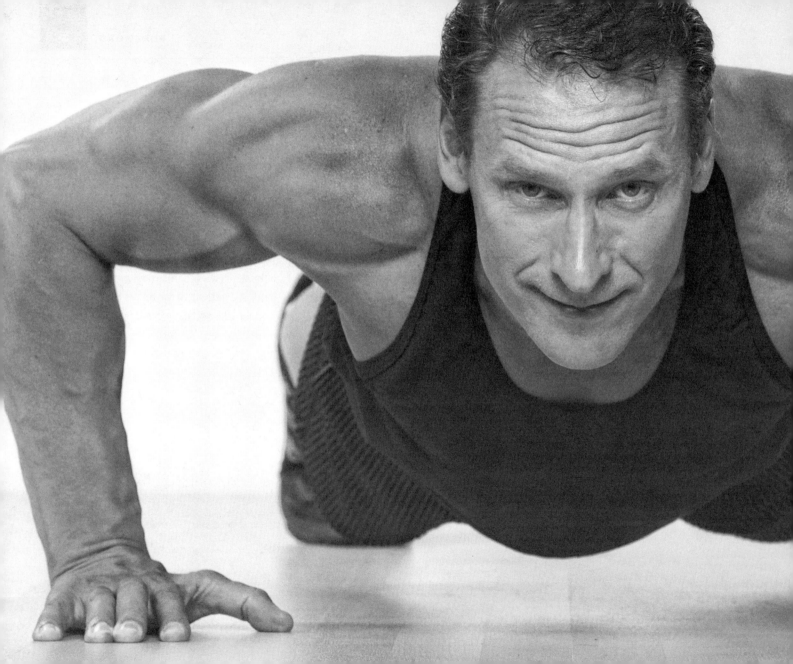

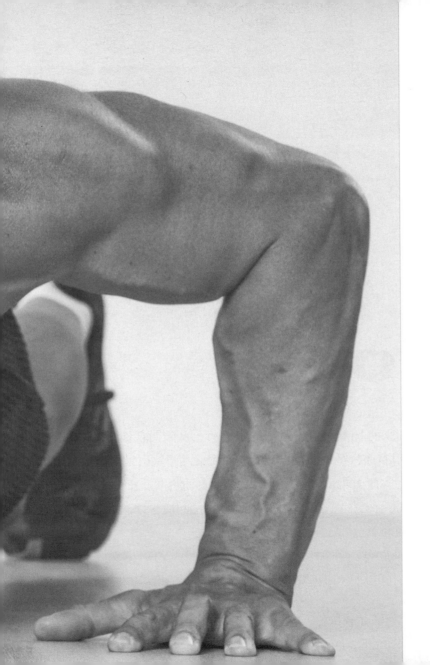

PART I:
OVERVIEW

Introduction

Hi, this is Brett. Thanks for picking up this book. Before you read another line, let's talk about the number 10, as in 10 pounds of muscle. It's a very specific number that may or may not jibe with your metabolism, athletic ability, or your body composition and ability to put on muscle. We chose 10 pounds as a high-end target based on the amount of muscle Jason and I were able to pack on in just under two months.

No, 10 pounds of muscle gain is not the end-all-be-all, and no one—other than you—is going to grade you on your success. Here's a little behind-the-scenes info: The original title of this muscle-building regimen was *7 Weeks to Getting BIG*, and the edit was made to provide a challenging and quantifiable target for the majority of athletes picking up this book for the first time.

Throughout this book you'll see references to things we've learned while testing the programs, stuff we've done right, and areas where we screwed up and needed to make changes. Why did we include all this? Because this book does not have the exact answer for how quickly your specific body will gain muscle; a one-size-fits-all program with a guarantee doesn't exist. Your DNA, not unlike your fingerprint, is yours and yours alone. Every function of your body from your heartbeat to your metabolism is unique to your own specific DNA fingerprint, and anyone who tells you that one certain method for developing muscle is best for you is full of shit. Plain and simple. If you don't believe me, then please put this book down and pick up one that purports that it has all the answers. Who knows, you might get lucky; more than likely you won't. If you're interested in learning about our approach and how it can help transform your body, then please read on.

Whether your goal is 5 or 15 pounds and your timeline is 7 weeks or 6 months, we've developed three different programs that can help you pack on muscle. Pick the one that's right for you and get to work. When combined with *7 Weeks to Getting Ripped*, our ultimate gym-free workout plan, these two programs can be a year-round alternating mass-building and definition regimen to get you in the best shape of your life!

How Did We Get Here?

JASON: I have a confession to make: I don't get paid to work out. No, fitness, working out and everything in between is a life obsession of mine, but no one pays me to do it. More confessions: The only people I've been ultra-jealous of in my life are those people who actually do get paid to work out. I'm talking professional athletes, actors and fitness models.

It all began when I started reading about the making of the movie *300* and how the actors and stuntmen went through a grueling six-month camp to get in movie shape. It. Sounded. Awesome. Instantly I was jealous. Imagine, getting paid (pretty well, I might add!) to work out. Get paid to have someone tell you what to do, to yell at you, to motivate you and to keep you on track. Get paid to have someone figure out the best food to eat and the proper time to eat it. Get paid to have someone build a custom routine and track it all for you. I can't imagine a better job in the world.

I've been obsessed with fitness ever since and it has paid me back with health, wellness, aesthetic muscles, improved athletic performance, discipline.

BRETT: Much like Jason, I would be completely geeked to get paid to work out or train constantly, but that's just not the case. When I became a certified personal trainer, I thought I would have the golden opportunity to work out alongside my clients on a daily basis, helping them achieve their fitness goals while getting into the best shape of my life. I found out quickly that was not the way personal training works. I was getting paid to focus strictly on my clients before, during and after workouts, and instead of working out along with them as I had done with countless training partners over the last decade, I had to carve out time to devote to my own fitness.

As a fitness author and full-time amateur athlete (is there such a thing?), being in shape for events of all shapes and sizes is a huge part of my life. Yet it always feels like I'm spinning my wheels when it comes to putting on muscle as I've never focused properly to make any significant gains. It has always seemed to me that Jason can simply look at a barbell and put on 10 pounds of muscle while I struggle to gain any mass. Does this make me a "hard gainer"? What does that term even really mean? (We'll cover the theory of body composition types, or somatotypes on page 36 in "What's My Body Type?")

Am I a hard gainer? Well, when I started this program I was absolutely convinced that I was—but I soon found out that I was wrong. Prior to testing this program, I had just never devoted myself to the time and effort of developing or following a specific regimen to pack on muscle. I can easily lose 5, 10, even 15 pounds when preparing for a marathon or triathlon because that's the type of training I put my effort into. In order to build the muscle I want, I need to focus on the proper training. There's no pill that will instantly make me a bulk-building machine nor is there a simple trick to making a new jacked-up physique possible without putting in the hard work required. The good news is there's a proven method for developing the most muscle in the shortest amount of time, provided you're willing to change everything about your workouts and nutrition: what you eat, when you eat, when you work out, how you work out. Your daily and weekly activities will get a bit of a shake-up, and—most importantly—your rest and sleep schedule will get a much-needed upgrade.

JASON: Shorter workouts. More food. More sleep. That surely can't be the quickest way to put on muscle, right? After all, we've been told that to get big you need to practically live in the gym and spend at least two to three hours lifting weights a day. But you'll be amazed at how quickly you can put on muscle by following a relatively simple protocol—I know I was! My results may not be typical, since I packed on over 22 pounds of muscle during the three-month test period. But I feel comfortable with using 10 pounds as a target for most folks following this 7-week program.

BRETT: I have no problem spending 15 to 20 hours a week running; that's something I'm good at. Bodyweight exercises, sprints, agility drills and most other high-octane exercises are right in my wheelhouse. I'm über-competitive when it comes to racing anything from 5Ks to marathons, triathlons and obstacle races or mud runs. I'm always up to the challenge for a trail run or even a 200-mile, 24-hour relay with 5 other guys. But lifting weights?

That's something I've just never been comfortable with. Frankly I've always had two fears: I've had some trepidation about hurting myself, dropping weights or looking like a fool in the gym.

Fear #1—Looking like a fool: As a 12-year-old kid, a pair of brothers in my neighborhood who were much bigger and stronger than I was laid out a challenge: If I could bench press the weight that was on their bar just once, they would let me ride their three-wheel motorbike. (Note: They stopped selling these things in the U.S. back in 1988, so that should give you a timeframe.) I didn't even bother counting up the weight and jumped right on the bench. How hard could one bench press be? Well, as the guys were lifting the bar off my chest amid my full-frenzied screaming panic, I realized I may have overestimated my strength. Good guys, those Perugini brothers, but 30-something years later I bet Bill and Mark still remember me crying like a baby to get that bar off of me in their garage. I also never did drive their three-wheeler.

Fear #2—Dropping weights in a gym: It wasn't until my late twenties that I ever touched a free weight bar on a bench again. Fifteen years had passed since the "garage incident," and the closest I'd ever come was a Nautilus machine and I had developed an actual phobia of being trapped by a weight while bench pressing. Chris Goggin (who I credit with kick-starting my fitness and endurance junkie addictions) conned me into joining

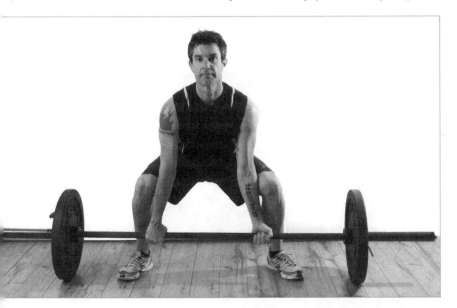

a gym with him and dutifully acted as my trainer and spotter. He helped me conquer my fear enough that a few weeks in I decided to finish my final set while he walked over to order a post-workout shake. At that moment, I was very proud of my confidence; 13 seconds later I was wondering how the heck I managed to push one side too high in order to make the bar uneven enough that a 45-pound plate would slide off and catapult the bar out of my hands in the opposite direction. While no one got hurt, the flying weights and bars and ensuing ruckus in a packed gym were absolutely humiliating—and marked one of the last times I showed my face in that gym (despite paying for membership for the next 8 months). If you have either of these fears see "Lifting Safely" on page 106.

The first time I ever even felt truly comfortable in a gym was when Jason and I were developing and testing the program in *7 Weeks to 50 Pull-Ups* and starting to create what would become the basis for *7 Weeks to Getting Ripped*. The reason for my new-found confidence was my ability to crank out more than 20 pull-ups in a row; at about 16 reps, a few other gym-goers would turn to see how long we'd keep going (Jason could usually do as many as I could too). After a few months of training three to five days a week at that gym and constantly developing new exercises, other members knew who we were and even started asking where the heck some of those moves like the hanging windshield wiper or J-up came from.

During one of our 100 burp-up (burpees plus pull-ups) challenges, Jason and I even had our own rooting section as we labored through an incredibly grueling event. The feedback and feeling of acceptance was extremely gratifying to a guy who never spent any time lifting free weights before. With Jason's help and patient guidance, I made the transition to learning Olympic lifts and eventually became well-rounded enough to grow as an athlete and over time honed my knowledge that led me to become a certified personal trainer.

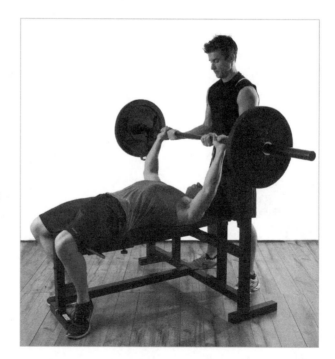

About the Book

This book has one focus: putting on muscle. In order to accomplish that goal, you'll have to follow a routine that will require you to eat, sleep and train differently than you ever have before. This book does not contain some mystical secret to packing on pounds of muscle mass without putting in the effort required, nor does it outline some hybrid program to develop speed or endurance. The entire scope of this book is to utilize a proven method of diet and exercises performed at specific times to maximize your body's ability to build muscle.

Any designs that you may have of developing a single-digit body fat percentage or shredding your torso to expose a six-pack need to be put on hold for now—because for the next 7 weeks you'll be developing your physique in ways you may never have thought possible and finally putting on real, solid muscle. *7 Weeks to 10 Pounds of Muscle* builds the most solid foundation possible for developing impressive strength, a chiseled physique, and improved athletic ability.

BRETT: Why this book? Simply put, at 42 years old, I wanted a new challenge to reshape my body and develop the bigger arms, chest, back and legs that I've never had. To put it bluntly, after almost a decade of running marathons, I'd grown sick and tired of checking the box "men's small T-shirt" on my race application. For the first time in my life, I wanted to fill out a large T-shirt with muscle—a bulging chest, bigger "guns" for arms, along with a broader upper back and shoulders. Now, I know 10 pounds is not going to transform me from looking like a triathlete to an MMA fighter, but it's surely a start!

Just as we did with *7 Weeks to Getting Ripped*, Jason and I were our own guinea pigs to research, develop and test the fitness and nutrition programs—with Corey's expert input, of course—and share the results with you in the easiest-to-follow manner. By the time we were through with testing, we were both confident that anyone who followed this plan would reap the benefits from the programs we'd put together. See "The Science behind It All" on page 75 for more in-depth information on how we created the exercise, rest, timing and nutritional protocols based on proven methods for rapidly developing lean muscle.

Everything about this plan was completely new to me, and this would be the first time I would attempt any program of this type. Lifting weights, changing my caloric intake, rebalancing my nutrition and this entirely different approach to training in general is a huge departure from my normal routine as a triathlete and marathoner and required a monumental shift in the way I looked at training, resting and eating. Honestly, my biggest difficulty was overcoming the obstacle between my ears. Wrapping my mind around eating more—much more—and exercising far less than I have been for nearly the last decade was a little bit strange to get used to and required me to refocus on building muscle versus burning fat. If I do say so myself, I'm really good at developing programs to lose weight, build speed and improve athletic performance; in order to take on this muscle-building program, I had to have faith that it would work. Luckily, my best friend Jason was the guy I had to put my faith in...and seeing as he was by my side while I trained for Ironman, ran alongside me during the Ragnar Del Sol ultramarathon relay and was my go-to guy for developing the *Ripped* program, it was a no-brainer.

JASON: Walk into any gym and look around. Notice the people, the styles of programs and what people are generally doing to achieve their goals. Fast forward 12 months, go back, see the same people. Chances are that the vast majority of people there (a) look the same, (b) lift the same weights or (c) all of the above, just as they did a year earlier. Clearly most people don't want to be on a fitness treadmill; rather, they would like to see visible improvement in their physique and physical improvement by moving more weights. But that's not what happens for most people in most circumstances; they remain relatively close to the same size and strength. Why is that?

Goals. Recognizing your goals and working to achieve them is vitally important. If your goal is to get in shape to run a marathon, you're reading the wrong book. If your goal is to run a 4.2-second 40-yard dash for the NFL combine, this book can potentially help you a tiny bit (having more muscle can't hurt), but it isn't optimized for that goal. However, if your goal is to look better naked and pack on some solid muscle, this is the book for you.

That's why this book. In all my time working out in gyms, nearly 90 percent of all men working out want to put on more muscle, yet they aren't working out or eating appropriately for that goal. And it really isn't their fault. Pick up any fitness magazine and you'll be inundated with "new" workouts, eating programs or routines that contradict each other, are inappropriate for the goal of putting on muscle or just don't work. But, if the so-called experts get it wrong, how is anyone going to know what to do? Hence, the workout treadmill. Year after year of not making progress. How frustrating.

We wrote this book to dispel myths, to provide a framework for success and, most of all, to outline a very definite way to achieve your goal of packing on muscle.

BRETT: Jason brings up a good point—*7 Weeks to 10 Pounds of Muscle* may be at the complete opposite of the spectrum from *7 Weeks to Getting Ripped*, but they both have the ability to complement each other to vastly overhaul your physique. In "Next Steps" on page 142, we cover a four- to six-month cycle using *Ripped* and *10 Pounds of Muscle* together to build the body of your dreams.

Why We Love Muscle

JASON: Performance, aesthetics, first impressions, evolutionary biology, primal instinct. Take your pick, I love muscle for all of the above. I love that it makes me better at sports, more attractive to the opposite sex, can create positive and lasting first impressions, not to mention that muscle plays into our evolutionary ancestry. Oh yeah, I love muscle, and I'm wagering so do you.

More importantly, we all love muscle. Society has an obsession with youth, vitality and musculature. We love our athletes to be hulking beasts performing inhuman acts that defy imagination and inspire awe. You can't make your way through a grocery store without seeing racks of shirtless people adorning magazine covers promising the secret to finally getting bigger and stronger.

BRETT: Because building muscle was always so elusive to me, I'd pretty much given up on the idea of getting bigger and focused on getting lean and becoming more competitive as an endurance athlete. I had set my physique up pretty well for marathons, notching my best time of 3:40 shortly after the release of *Ripped*, and it wasn't until I was doing all the research for *Ultimate Obstacle Race Training: Crush the World's Toughest Courses* that I got really serious about building the upper-body strength I needed to lift, carry and drag stuff much heavier than I was used to. It wasn't long after my first Spartan Race that I realized that while I was fit and could run circles around a lot of other competitors, I could use an upgrade in my musculature to finish a lot faster and potentially get to the podium. I'm ultra-competitive, and falling short is not something I felt comfortable with. In order to hit my new goals, I needed to embrace change and come at my training from a new angle.

JASON: If we love rippling muscles and covet them for ourselves, why is there so much confusion over how to get them? A much better questions is: Why are there so many confusing and contradictory programs published each month in various fitness magazines? More often than not, men's or women's fitness magazines will feature diametrically opposed workouts in the same issue!

BRETT: The simple answer? We're all responsible for letting them get away with it by purchasing these magazines full of somewhat confusing or contradictory exercise routines. The more shocking answer is because each of these articles, exercise programs or nutritional regimens are actually right—provided they match up perfectly with your goals and ability. Nearly any workout or diet has the ability to be ideal for any individual. Let me restate that: Almost any fitness or nutritional regimen has the ability to deliver the results you are looking for, provided the program's goals match up with the results you are seeking:

- weight loss
- toning
- muscle gain
- endurance
- speed
- flexibility
- enhanced athletic performance

Even if they do match your goals, for you to be successful in sticking with this regimen for the duration, you'll require that the:

- physical routine is within your ability level;

- exercises and programs are relatively simple to repeat and keep you engaged for the entire duration;

- routine is sustainable for at least three months, reducing the chance of unhealthy yo-yo weight loss and gain, as well as short, rapid weight loss through extreme measures;

- foundation is built on actual science, physiology and kinesiology;

- "diet" is sound, and not some fad. Rapid-weight-loss pills, cleanses, juices, extreme calorie restrictions or meal replacements are potentially dangerous and potentially only deliver short-term benefits followed by immediate weight gain;

Prior to writing *7 Weeks to Getting Ripped*, I was positive that Jason and I had developed the ultimate workout that anyone could use for all-around perfect fitness, and that this pinnacle of fitness could be achieved through bodyweight workouts improving strength, agility, speed and endurance. Over a year of experience, hundreds of thousands of hits to the *Ripped* program online and thousands of e-mails, tweets, Facebook posts and face-to-face conversations later, I realized that while we had created a program that has dramatically improved athletic performance and physiques of countless individuals worldwide, we didn't cover a wide enough spectrum of goals. Requests were pouring in for recommendations to pack on large amounts of muscle while using the familiar, repeatable and sound exercises found in *Ripped*. After months of research and testing, we came to the realization that this new goal was relatively impossible. You see, the goals of *Getting Ripped* are to deliver strength, speed, agility, weight loss and overall fitness through cross-training, yet aren't a perfect fit for the average athlete that wants to pack on as much lean muscle in as little time as possible.

Ripped was created with the following mindset: If we were to ask trainers all over the globe what their clients hire them for, the answers fall into what we'd like to call our top-three categories:

Get off your ass-ivation: Using a trainer for motivation, supervision and to provide some accountability to keep the individual on track for general fitness, health and longevity. "I paid my trainer for 12 sessions, so I need to show up" can be the deciding factor for individuals to continue working out. Whatever it takes, right?

Get rid of my ass-ivation: Weight loss and toning, usually for a life event like a wedding, beach vacation, class reunion or new-found single status forcing you to look somewhat presentable to the opposite sex. "Boot camps" are really popular with this group because they're usually looking for immediate results.

Move your ass-ivation: Athletic improvement or sport-specific training for an upcoming season or events. Speed, core strength, endurance and flexibility are a common focus for most sports that involve getting

THE BASICS OF MUSCLES

The *7 Weeks to 10 Pounds of Muscle* program is based on four main lifts: deadlift, barbell press, overhead press and squat. Those exercises together work all the body's major muscle groups.

The deadlift works both the upper and lower body, as well as the back: the gluteus maximus (glutes), hamstrings and back muscles, including the latissimus dorsi (lats), trapezius (traps) and rhomboids, are the main movers; the quadriceps (quads) also get some work, as do the deltoids.

In the overhead press, the main muscles recruited are the latissimus dorsi, deltoids and triceps, but you should also feel some work in the pectorals (pecs), rhomboids, core, gluteus maximus and quadriceps.

Barbell squats blast the entire lower body, working your quadriceps, hamstrings, gluteus maximus and hip flexors all at once. Your core also gets blasted, and your upper back is used for stabilizing the bar.

The barbell press uses the pectorals, shoulders, triceps, biceps and core. This means you're pumping up those vanity muscles: chest and arms.

So where are all these muscles on your body? Check out page 20 for a rundown on what's what.

from point A to point B as rapidly as possible, especially athletic endeavors where you repeat that over and over (e.g., soccer, football, baseball, paintball, etc.).

Usually a specific target of putting on "X pounds of muscle in X amount of time" isn't on the tip of a client's tongue when they're asked what their training goals are, although it appears to be on their minds. Just Google "putting on muscle," sift through the 69 million results, and you'll realize how important packing on solid, lean muscle is to athletes worldwide.

Now, those top-three "ass-ivation" goals above aren't mutually exclusive; you can lose weight, get healthy, improve your athletic ability and develop a fantastic physique all at the same time. Heck, that's what *7 Weeks to Getting Ripped* was created for. But when it comes to packing on pounds of muscle, that requires a different approach to workouts, rest and nutrition that almost fly directly in the face of the *Ripped* protocols; you'll be working out for shorter periods of time with heavier weights, eating more and resting a lot more to reach your goals.

JASON: The goals of *Ripped* could be described as five knobs: speed, endurance, strength, physique and overall athletic performance. To hit the goals you want when using that program, you can dial in each of those knobs according to your intensity, ability and how each knob relates to your desired results. If you're working toward a 10K personal best, you may crank the virtual

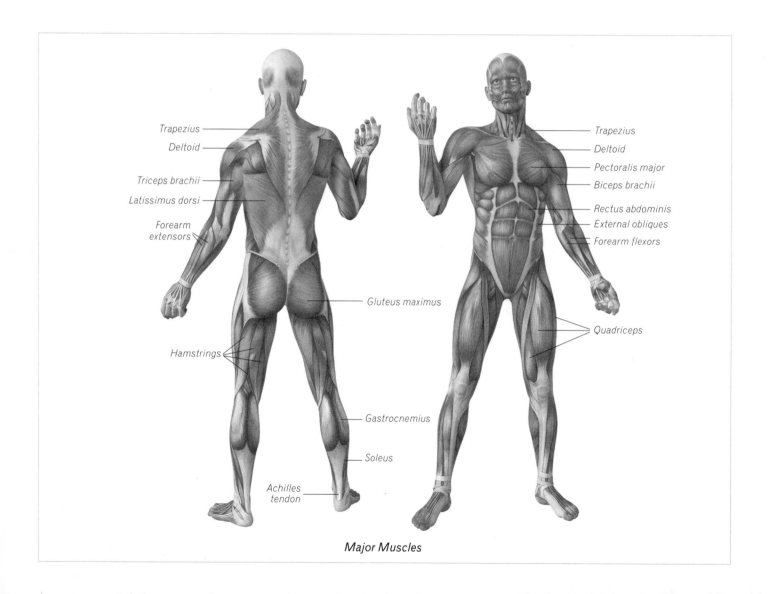

Major Muscles

speed knob up to 10 and mentally set the strength dial at a 4. For those who want to look their best, they would focus on physique most, right?

7 Pounds to 10 Pounds of Muscle only has one knob, period. If you're committed to packing on serious muscle in under two months, you need to focus on one goal and one goal only: developing solid, lean muscle. This book is not titled *Get Six-Pack Abs while Building Huge Biceps* nor is it *Run a Marathon while Developing a Body of Steel*; this book is dedicated to the singular pursuit of packing on healthy muscle. You've got to commit to the process and subscribe to the workouts, rest and nutrition if you want to see the results. Half-assing this routine is the quickest way to fail.

BRETT: I initially had some doubts about jumping into the program. Since Jason and I always put our money where our mouth is, we had to put ourselves through the program in order to see which parts work, find areas that need tweaking and make sense of all the lessons we'd learn along the way. As a "model" in several fitness books, my physique gets scrutinized by readers. I've received a few e-mails chiding me for my flabby appearance in *7 Weeks to 50 Pull-Ups*, but many more commending me for being a "normal guy" working hard to get—and stay—fit. Readers have followed my progression and body transformation from one book to the next, and stepping up to the plate to pack 10 pounds

of muscle on my 42-year-old runner's frame took a bit of prodding from Jason and a bit of relinquishing control on my end. In order to follow the program, I would change my training drastically from the constant running and bodyweight routines that have been a huge part of my life for nearly the last decade and get outside my comfort zone with weights, eating a lot more (healthy) calories and reducing my running regimen nearly to zero. By week three, any doubts I had of the program's effectiveness were erased, and with the addition of Corey's Muscle-Building Nutrition Plan, my wife and friends began to notice the growth of my biceps, chest and upper back less than halfway through the 7 weeks.

JASON: Brett brings up another great point— where would this book be without Corey? How effective could a muscle-building book be without a sensible, easy-to-follow nutritional plan to help you build healthy mass while having the energy to perform each workout?

BRETT: In a word? Nowhere. Lifting, eating and sleeping are the three important elements in this program, and without Corey's nutritional strategy, this book would have a rudimentary chapter on "stuff we eat" rather than a comprehensive plan. If it weren't for Corey's input, I'd be eating eggs and chicken breast all day, every day. Over seven weeks, that would probably lead to me hating those foods for the rest of my life. There's no doubt Jason and I needed a professional chef, fitness coach and input from a nutritionist to hit our goals, and without question this book gains a significant amount of class by having her on board.

COREY: Thanks, guys! Yes, we certainly want to give people lots of food choices so they enjoy their food and stay interested in what they're eating while they're packing on the muscle. As a chef and a coach, I look at food as both fuel and fun. High-performance eating can and should be a pleasurable experience, because that means that athletes will be more likely to stick with the program. There's no doubt about it—a targeted, performance-oriented eating program, when paired with an effective exercise program, breeds results. This is why the food selections are varied and have been specifically tailored to meet the goals of this book. And, just like the exercises, the recipes and the meal plan have been personally tested by Jason, Brett and me. In fact, I eat everything I make, and so do my family and friends. Believe me, that's a lot of collective, useful feedback, as the lot of them are athletes. While I was creating the nutritional program, the input I received from Brett and Jason was invaluable, because while you've got to build muscle in the gym and the kitchen, one is useless without the other; they have to complement each other for maximum effectiveness. I've even been inspired by Brett and Jason to start lifting more weight in the gym. After all, we ladies want to look buff too.

Our Approach

No one knows exactly how muscle grows for every single individual. There are theories, plenty of anecdotal evidence and massive amounts of the aforementioned gym science, but we don't know exactly the biological mechanisms, environmental situations and hormonal balances that produce the optimal situation to grow muscle for every person. What works for Jason doesn't necessarily have the same effect on Brett. We do know elements. It takes testosterone, insulin, stress and recovery. We know that certain actions cause more muscle growth than others. For instance, lifting heavy weights makes muscles grow while running does not.

But the exact formula, we don't have it. The science just isn't there. This leads to quite a bit of contradictory theories and "experts" giving very conflicting advice. This is also how we end up with people advising completely different training programs all designed to build muscle. What are you to do when one expert says you need a heavy-weight, low-rep, low-volume program, another says you need a moderate-weight, high-rep, high-volume program and still another says the only sensible approach is a program based around tension?

However, that doesn't mean we don't know anything. On the contrary, there are things we know and can use to hack the body. First, we know that it takes stress and overloading the body to achieve results. Second, we know the body needs time to recover from the stress. And third, we know that certain food choices and food times create a more beneficial environment for muscle growth. We are going to dispel the myths, give a sensible program taking the best of all the approaches and provide a foolproof way to pack on solid quality muscle.

The basic program styles we'll lay bare are three things: progressive resistance (strength training), increasing volume (volume training) and constant muscular tension (tension training). Further, we have some basic principles that guide us every day when we are in the gym.

Under the Bar

To build solid, lifelong muscle, you need to be "under the bar," and by this we mean you need to find yourself a 45-pound Olympic straight bar and get yourself underneath it! There are four basic lifts that will become your new best friends: flat-bar bench press, overhead press, deadlift and barbell squat.

These lifts will form the basis for the program in this book and will be featured on a given day along with some supporting exercises. These four basic lifts combined

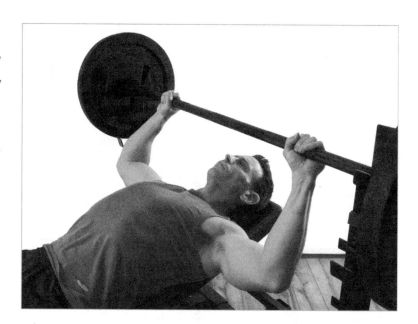

work your entire body in a way substitutions just can't. People generally hate squats and want to incorporate easier leg exercises, to which we just say NO. There's a reason people stay away from those lifts: They're hard. And they're hard for a reason. They are tried-and-true exercises that work your body in ways the substitutions do not. And, after all, the whole point of this program is to get the maximum you can out of your body!

Everything Is Relative

This program is all relative to you. The weights you will be lifting from your first set to your last are based on *your* ability—not the authors', not your training partner's nor anyone else in the gym. You're building your body based on ratcheting up your maximum lifts from workout to workout and need to get it out of your head that you should be lifting the same amount as anyone else. There will always be others lifting more weight in the gym— get over it. You're here to build you, not to worry about impressing them.

Let's put it this way, Brett started this program at 148 pounds, while Jason tipped the scales at 216. Do you think there's any shot that both these guys would max out at the same weight? Relatively speaking, they may be lifting, pushing and pressing close to the same amount of weight relative to their own body weight, but as each individual has different strengths and weaknesses, some lifts will be easier and allow you to lift more while some may force you to use lighter weights to maintain proper form. The most important part is that you focus on lifting a weight that is as heavy as possible while allowing you to complete all your target reps for each movement and progressing to incrementally heavier weights with each successive workout. We refer to this progression as "Beat the Book."

Beat the Book

Read any workout regimen, blog or book on getting stronger and you'll see quite a bit of talk about reps, sets and optimal rep ranges. There's quite a bit of study on the subject but not a lot of conclusive evidence one way or another. There's plenty of overlapping and contradictory "gym science" relating to what's optimal, and everyone is left to decipher all this on their own. How is this book different? For one thing, we spent plenty of time researching and testing some of the different protocols and learned as much as we could about the ins and outs. Then, we adapted as many of the useful pieces as possible and developed a blended approach that combines the principles of progressive overloading, increasing volume and time under tension—the three most effective ways to build muscle, fast.

Put your confusion and fears aside: packing on muscle doesn't need to be so damn frustrating. Instead, we're going to keep it as simple as we possibly can. No complicated rules to follow, just some guidelines. This one is called "Beat the Book." It simply means that with each workout you should be improving in some way, whether that be going up in reps, weight or volume—just improve. How you improve is going to be subject to how you feel. Feel like you can handle more weight? Do the same reps and sets as the last workout but with more weight. Are the weights feeling heavy today? Do the same weight and reps for an extra set, or the same sets and weights but for more reps.

The basic point is that you want to be moving forward, lifting progressively heavier weights and increasing the volume and increasing the time the muscle is working generally, in that order.

Maxing Your T

Why do you want testosterone? Aside from increased energy, sex drive, improved memory and focus, testosterone (or T) is responsible for the body's ability to gain and maintain lean muscle mass in men and women. While women normally have only about 10 percent the level of testosterone men do, it's just as vital for them to maintain that level of this hormone. Testosterone production in your muscles is a vicious circle (a viciously awesome one) where the more lean muscle you pack on your body, the more lean muscle you can build... which in turn allows for those muscles to pump out even more T. The old adage "It takes money to make money" could easily be applied here; just swap out money for testosterone. Maxing out your testosterone—naturally—is the key to building lean muscle, improving your physique, raising your energy levels and feeling more focused and happier all-around.

Unfortunately, there are several factors at play to actually reduce your testosterone production:

Getting older (hey, it happens to us all). Starting at age 30, testosterone production begins to drop by 1–2% per year. Scary, huh?

Falling in love and having children. Seriously! Research has shown a male T reduction in the first 1–3 years of a committed relationship as well as becoming a father. Women's bodies actually increase testosterone during the onset of a relationship, and have a pretty complicated testosterone/estrogen balance during pregnancy and after childbirth; we're not going into that here.

Gaining weight. Lean muscle produces testosterone, fatty tissue produces estrogen, the anti-T.

There are other, more serious ways to diminish your T (serious illness, treatments such as chemotherapy, wasting diseases, etc.), but let's start with ones that we all can recognize. You can't control the first one above at all, and there's a pretty darn good chance you won't pass up the second one either. But the third is totally doable!

Testosterone deficiency can rob a man or woman of their mojo. It can cause diminished sex drive, low energy and a general feeling of malaise, and lead to much more serious conditions such as obesity, brittle bones, muscle loss and impotence. To make matters much worse, you increase your chance of dying of a heart attack. Normal levels of testosterone in a male vary from 270 up to 1,070 nanograms per deciliter (ng/dl), women 15 to 70. T levels below or at the lower end of that spectrum increase your risks of the problems listed above; your body just isn't producing enough and you're becoming, or already are, testosterone-deficient.

No section on testosterone would be complete without mentioning "getting on the juice" or injecting testosterone to boost your performance, so let's give it a cursory overview.

First off, if you believe you have seriously low levels of testosterone because of diminished sex drive or energy, see a doctor for a simple blood test to check your androgen level. Why? Because even if swallowing T-boosting pills, rubbing on androgen-raising topical creams or sticking on a testosterone patch will increase your T, that may not be the right therapy for you! Problems with your pituitary or adrenal glands, testicles or ovaries demand serious attention from a licensed physician, not a hook-up from a buddy who knows where you can get the "good stuff." Testosterone therapy should only be done under the supervision of a trained, competent physician who takes all of your health factors into account; don't screw with this stuff yourself, relying on information from the Internet or someone who claims "it worked for them." Messing with your hormones is not something to take lightly. Professional athletes who've been caught for doping have been shown to have very highly paid medical professionals (with questionable ethics) assisting them. Even with all that assistance, they're playing with fire by screwing around—and possibly screwing up—the only body that they'll ever have.

Luckily, you can kick-start natural production of this powerhouse hormone you want to maximize by doing some or all of the following:

- **Drop the flab.** Excess fat elevates estrogen levels, causing testosterone production to become limited.

- **Eat well.** A balanced diet with the proper amount of protein, carbs and fat each day will maximize your production; a severe overload on protein and removing all carbs can actually inhibit T production.

- **Have more sex.** What can we say, it does a body good!

- **Multi-joint, multi-muscle lifts.** Squat, bench press, deadlift and overhead press are staples of the *7 Weeks to 10 Pounds of Muscle* program for very good reason. Compound exercises train multiple large muscle groups—the more muscle mass at work, the more testosterone released. Follow the reps, style and weight recommendations in the program for maximal results.

- **Limit alcohol consumption.** Too much booze not only affects sex drive and performance, it also screws with your body's ability to produce testosterone and process nutrients from your food, and sabotages your judgment...'nuff said.

- **Get more quality sleep.** More REM sleep, more often. Your muscles need time to rest, heal, recover and grow. Check out "Rest Is Not for Sissies," page 30, where we cover some tips to get better sleep.

- **Don't overtrain.** Never hit the same muscle groups day after day. Not only are you limiting your muscle's ability to heal and grow by continually putting it under stress, overtraining can choke off circulating testosterone levels by as much as 35%. You're not doing yourself any favors by hitting the same muscles day after day, you're sabotaging yourself.

Testosterone helps to raise your metabolism, torch body fat and promote lean muscle gain. In turn, that lean muscle requires more energy and continues to stoke your body's metabolic fire, which promotes weight loss. You'll simply burn more calories with your excess lean muscle because it's an active tissue that requires cellular repair and maintenance, blood flow, etc. It's pretty easy to see how maximizing your natural T will help you maximize your body's true potential and one heckuva lean, muscular physique.

Insulin's Role in Bigger Muscles

Insulin is produced by the pancreas and released when carbohydrates (glucose) and proteins enter the bloodstream. Its primary function is to regulate blood sugar levels by increasing glucose uptake and storage in the liver, muscle and fat tissue. The stored glucose can then be used as an energy source when blood sugar levels drop. While insulin's role in the body is extremely important for us all to function, it can be a double-edged sword when building muscle and re-shaping your physique. Below is a simplified overview of how insulin regulates your metabolic systems and aids in tissue-building. For more in-depth resources on insulin, check out www.7weekstofitness.com for some research links.

The negative aspect of insulin for those looking to pack on lean muscle is that the release of insulin from the pancreas immediately stops the body from burning fat as an energy source. A layer of fat is really going to compromise that muscle definition, right? See, while you're sleeping, magic little fairies sprinkle fat-burning dust into your snoring maw to ignite your metabolism and turn you into an efficient fat-melting machine. Not buying the fairies? OK, an overly simplified description of what really happens is during your overnight fast while your body's systems are running on low power (think of energy-save mode on your laptop) and you've used up all the glycogen in your blood for energy, your metabolic system switches over to burning fat to keep all systems functioning. Even when you wake up, fat burning is still happening at an elevated level, and it's not until you ingest that first morsel of food containing carbohydrates or protein that insulin is released and your body flips the switch back to burning glycogen—and that fat-burning advantage is gone. We'll talk more about timing and how to elongate this window of fat-burning to your advantage in Part III.

On the positive side, insulin can be responsible for helping your body build bigger muscles due to its anabolic effect. It enhances protein synthesis and amino acid uptake to muscle cells, and it increases blood flow to aid in faster muscle cell repair and growth—all stuff you want to happen when you're trying to pack on lean muscle. Insulin also inhibits the catabolization of your protein, which just means that it saves your muscles' prime source of growth from being converted to energy and burned by the body as fuel. Finally, the blood flow that insulin facilitates also facilitates glycogen storage in muscle cells, resulting in much fuller, denser muscles.

How do you get all the benefits of insulin without all the bad? It's really not that hard, but it will take some discipline and proper timing on your part, especially when you introduce carbohydrates into your body. We'll cover this all in much more depth in the nutrition section, though the highlights are quite easy to grok:

1. Carb timing is critically important. Carbs are for building muscle, so you should eat them after working out.
2. Before you workout, your body isn't ready for carbs. Introducing carbs when your body is not ready basically signals it to store fat. Do not do this.
3. High-GI carbs are OK post-workout. Low-GI carbs are a safe bet whenever you reach for a carb source.
4. Unless you're special (hint: you aren't), don't combine fat and carbs. Bad things happen with both of those are in your body at the same time.

Pace Yourself

The following phrase should come as no big surprise: Building muscle is hard. For the most part, building solid, lean muscle is much harder than losing fat. What we're giving you here is the culmination of years of research, experimentation and advancement. Even so, it's going to take work, discipline and, most importantly, time.

Do not, repeat, DO NOT develop workout ADD. This is when you start to get a bit bored, or think you aren't seeing the results you wanted to see fast enough and decide to "shake it up" and change your workout, your diet or both at the same time. Stick with the program, see it through to the end and you'll be quite pleased with the results.

BRETT: This is my "workout kryptonite" no matter what I'm training for—triathlons, marathons, getting ready for a photo shoot or even during the initial testing for this program. I suck at sticking to a program because I feel constrained by the restricted regimen or get bored with repeating the same series of workouts. There's always something else I should be doing or trying out this new program or that one; look, over there—a shiny object! Once we nailed down the Advanced version of this program and I got 100 percent on-board with the exercises, I found my workouts flying by and the weeks ticking off more quickly than I'd expected. Every time I felt like straying (or signing up to run a trail marathon)

I'd focus on the gains I was making. I signed on for seven weeks to build muscle and reshape my body. Less than halfway through, I was filling out a T-shirt much better than when I'd started, and the only way to get the results I wanted was to stick to the program. So, I did!

Rest Is Not for Sissies

When does your muscle grow? In the gym or outside the gym? An easy question to answer, but harder to put into practice. Of course your muscle grows when you're not in the gym. Technically it mostly repairs itself when you're sleeping. Take the naps, get 8 hours of sleep a night and make sure you get adequate rest between workouts. The program will call for 4 workout days and 3 rest days. USE ALL THE REST DAYS! Do not be tempted to "just work out a little" on those days. Give your body time to heal. We're going to be throwing quite a bit at you pretty quickly. Take advantage of all the time off allotted.

JASON: Lately I've seen more articles and studies on the topic of athletes realizing the importance of sleep and utilizing high-tech, expensive beds to maximize the effectiveness of their sleep by getting the most REM sleep possible. While you may not have the budget as professional athletes, you can benefit from some of the same tips they use:

- **Get at least 8 hours of sleep every night.** That includes weekends too. Your circadian rhythms are easily knocked off-balance by late-night partying (or book writing).

- **Minimize any exercise or activity within one hour of bed.** By the time you hop into the sack your heart rate should be at a resting level.

- **Turn off your electronic devices.** Living rooms are for TVs, bedrooms are (mostly) for sleep. Leave your mobile device, laptop or tablet in the other room; lit-up screens have been shown to disrupt early sleep patterns and keep you from falling asleep quickly. Falling asleep with the TV on generally means you'll stay up far later than you intended and only nod off when the infomercials start airing, right?

- **Turn off your brain too.** Your bedroom should be a peaceful, relaxing sanctuary where you sleep and escape from all your stresses. Worrying does not promote a restful state, and you most likely won't fix your issues while you're in bed. Maximize your mattress-time effectively by getting quality sleep.

- **Set the scene for rest.** Keep your room dark with heavy curtains to block as much light as possible and use a fan or noise machine to provide a soothing sound to lull you to sleep.

- **Fuel your body to build muscle during sleepy-time.** Protein provides the critical amino acids that serve as building blocks for the formation of new muscle. Casein and whey are the two non-soy protein powders you'll find at nearly any grocery or health-food store. While whey is metabolized quickly and should be taken immediately after a workout, casein protein is metabolized slowly and perfect for keeping your body anabolic while you're asleep.

Grow Now, Shred Later

Cardio takes a backseat when you're lifting to gain muscle. Every drop of energy needs to be going into repairing the microtears in your muscles and rebuilding your muscles bigger than they were before. Now, we're not saying you need to be completely inactive outside of your lifting regimen, just make sure to take in even more calories to replace those you've lost and really try to maximize your rest periods. If you're only getting 6 hours (or less) of sleep and then heading out for a run on an empty tank, then you're simply not focusing on building muscle at an accelerated rate through this program. Seven weeks isn't a long time to commit yourself to building muscle. You'll have plenty of time to get ripped later, and we'll even show you how to do it!

BRETT: "Hi, my name is Brett, and I'm a runner. It's been three weeks since my last set of intervals...." I had to ditch my daily obsession of trail running and scale back on my mileage significantly in order to take this program seriously. Yes, it was a little difficult to let my racing shoes catch dust for weeks at a time, but at least I had the daily dog walks and an occasional jog to clear my head (if not, my wife would have most likely killed me), and I kept playing in my coed and men's soccer leagues. I try to live up to my "Tenacious" nickname, and once I locked in on my goal of building muscle, I knew I'd have to forgo running for a bit, and I'm really happy I did. Not coincidentally, my hips, quads, calves and hamstrings were stronger after 7 weeks and after shaking some of the rust off I was running more quickly with a few new PRs (personal records) to boot.

K.I.S.S. (Keep It Simple, Stupid)

People make lifting weights too complicated. At its core, it is really simple: Lift as heavy a thing as you can as many times as you can. Repeat.

Of course, proper form is critical to building muscle without injury, but form doesn't matter if you're too overwhelmed by all the "do this and don't do that" that accompanies a lot of complicated workouts. If you're too confused by a program to get off your ass and go to the gym, then you've clearly picked up the right book this

time. Without a ton of mumbo-jumbo and a decent dose of common sense, we'll provide a workout that is simple in form and easy to remember and repeat.

This program aims to K.I.S.S. for both the workout and diet portions. Step-by-step instructions, easy-to-follow guidelines and just a few principles. These guidelines and principles will last a lifetime and allow you many years of happy muscle building.

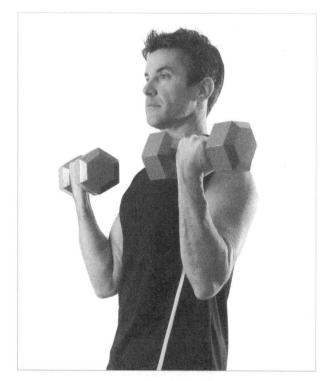

Frequently Asked Questions

Q. What's the hardest part of following this program?

A. Eating, eating and eating. Adding around 2,000 or more calories a day to your diet can be difficult. That's probably a lot more food than you're used to consuming every day!

Q. How long is this going to take me, really?

A. It depends on your goals, your drive, your metabolism...and a whole other host of factors (age, sex, testosterone level, muscular imbalances, training ability), not to mention the most important factor—having a life.

Q. If I follow along, am I guaranteed to pack on 10 pounds of muscle in 7 weeks?

A. There are no guarantees in life, and this program is no exception. We can personally guarantee that you will not gain exactly 10 pounds. Period. This is not a "one size fits all" program, and you'll have to take the advice and programs and make tweaks to fit your body and timing adjustments to fit your life, all the while remembering that all the weights are relative to your strength and ability. If you start this program with three of your friends, expect four slightly different results. All of the results should be extremely positive, but if you're worried about gaining the exact number of ounces of muscle as your buddy, then you're worrying about the wrong thing. Focus on your results, maximize the program for your ability and you'll be pleased with the results.

Q. Can I do this?

A. Is it doable? Absolutely. Both Brett and Jason both proudly smashed their personal goals, overcame plenty of mistakes and missteps, and continued to tweak the program to get positive results and surpass what they expected to accomplish. You can too.

Q. Can I just build bigger biceps using this program?

A. No, this is a full-body program, not designed to target any particular muscle group. You'll get bigger arm, leg and chest muscles, and whatever overall gains you make will be spread over your entire physique.

Q. My friend told me that you should only/never/always do this or that and he's huge!

A. Good for him, we're wicked psyched that he's huge. You have a bazillion choices for workout routines, there is no "perfect program" that fits everyone. Be sure to ask him how he researched his program, how long it took, how hard he trains, what and when he eats, what sacrifices he had to make and all the things he did wrong along the way. Or you can get that insight from us right here. Will our routines and his be exactly the same? Absolutely not. Will ours work for you if you put in the effort and follow it? You betcha.

Q. I've got a bad knee/shoulder/elbow/hip. Can I still follow the program?

A. Have you seen your doctor? No, seriously—go see your doctor before you start any fitness or nutrition program. Since you'll be lifting heavy weights, it'll be important for you to have as much full range of motion, a stable base and balance in your musculature as possible. A ripped ACL will greatly affect your ability to perform heavy squats, and a rotator cuff injury will surely hinder presses, rows...you get the idea. While we provide some alternate exercises, injuries are surely going to hamper your ability to perform certain movements. Be smart, lift within your ability and let injuries heal before pushing too hard. You're going to have this body for the rest of your life—there's plenty of time to recover and pack on muscle when you're ready.

NOTE: If you skip squats and deadlifts, you're limiting your ability to pack on muscle. It's just the facts; multi-joint exercises are a big part of the mass-building protocol.

Q. I've seen other muscle-building programs. How does this differ?

A. These programs provide a linear approach to training, offering people programs that they can use their entire life. These programs also combine the approaches that make other programs successful and reject the fluff that causes frustration. Simply put, this is as cutting edge as it gets for hypertrophy programming.

Q. Can I jump right to Intermediate or Advanced?

A. Generally, no, you should not. However, we offer this. If you've been working out for some time and can squat 1.5 times your weight, deadlift 2 times your weight and

bench press 1.25 times your weight, even though we would still want you to go through the Prep program, you have achieved decent enough numbers in the core lifts that we feel comfortable enough for you to start with Intermediate.

No one should jump to Advanced regardless. Everyone should at least go through the Intermediate program.

Q. If volume is better than strength for pure muscle size, shouldn't I do more volume and less strength training?

A. Science test: Which builds more muscle—a single 600-pound bench press or a 1-pound bench press 600 times? The answer? Obviously the 600-pound bench press is more taxing on the system. But the truth is we don't know where the line is drawn on the spectrum. Is a 20-rep 100-pound bench press more beneficial than a 5-rep 300-pound bench press?

What do we know? That more volume is good, but more volume at higher weights is better. We know that you can't lift heavier weights without being stronger.

Another very unscientific way of looking at this is just by asking the question: Have you ever seen a small person able to bench press 400 pounds, squat 500 pounds or deadlift 600 pounds? Neither have we.

The fact is that being strong is generally beneficial to gaining muscle in several ways, none more so to the goal of lifting heavier weights at a higher volume. If you can

WHAT'S MY BODY TYPE?

Are you destined to fail when trying to gain muscle? Are the cards stacked against you when it comes to genetics and you just can't develop muscle at the same rate as your buddies or that guy on the fitness magazine cover? Should you just throw in the towel now because you're not built like an Adonis with a broad back and shoulders?

First and foremost, your results are YOUR RESULTS. Unless you're planning for a pose-down on stage for a bodybuilding contest, it simply does not matter what everyone else around you looks like, trains like or how much they can lift. That dude's bulging biceps should mean nothing to you or how you should train your body.

In order to dispel some myths about what perceived limitations each person's musculature may contain, it is important to briefly explain theories of somatotypes, classifications of the human physique as purported by William H. Sheldon during his studies in the 1940s, followed by his book *Atlas of Men* in 1954. Intended to describe the physical traits of all humans—size, shape and musculature—as well as each type's ability to build muscle or gain fat, Sheldon's classifications are:

- Ectomorphic: long and thin muscles/limbs and low fat storage; usually referred to as slim. Not predisposed to store fat or build muscle.
- Mesomorphic: medium bones, solid torso, low fat levels, wide shoulders with a narrow waist; usually referred to as muscular. Predisposed to build muscle but not store fat.
- Endomorphic: characterized by increased fat storage, a wide waist, and large bone structure. Often referred to as "stocky" or "round," with short thick necks and limbs and a relatively soft-looking physique.

You'll still hear those terms used today, but take them with a grain of salt. With training, weight loss (or gain) and body re-composition (packing on muscle), most individuals fall into the pseudo-classification "gray area." To sum it up with one simple phrase: Don't get too hung up on it. We can't even tell you what classification we each fall into, but each of us straddles more than one.

bench press 100 pounds 20 times, wouldn't you assume that 200 pounds 20 times is better? Hint: It is. And how do you get to this? By building your strength.

Q. My buddy at the gym got great results from X, Y or Z. Why isn't that in this program?

A. There are many things excluded from this program that are actually useful in the right setting. For instance, partial reps, deficit lifts and negative reps are great ways for advanced lifters to achieve specific results. However, they are great for specific reasons, and those reasons

aren't the main goal of this book. When you achieve a level of understanding of the various programming protocols and your own body, and your strength numbers are high enough, you can feel free to experiment with these. In the meantime, follow this program and eat big and you'll achieve more than you ever thought you could more quickly than you thought possible.

Q. Do I really need to do 5–8 seconds down for tension training?

A. Yes, this is a critical aspect to getting the most out of your muscles for that training style. To prove to yourself that this does indeed work, let's do a quick experiment. I want you to drop and do 1 push-up, right now. But I want you to make the push-up last 1 minute in total: 30 seconds down and 30 seconds up. How do you feel? Thought so.

Q. But all those guys bouncing the weights and using modified or improper form are still getting results. What gives?

A. Nearly any training program will get results for some period of time. That is the nature of the body. However, they are putting their joints under more stress for basically nothing. The same results can be achieved using lighter weights and slower, more precise movements. And as we noted, lifting heavy weights does do something magical for the body, we just combined all the approaches to get the optimal results. Resist the urge to bounce those weights! Do not use momentum and gravity...fight it!

To prove why this is important, another experiment. This one might be harder to do, though we do encourage you to try. Find a big truck and three or four friends. Put the truck in neutral and try to push it. Most likely you can't. Get your friends to help, but as soon as it's moving, have them stop and you continue. More than likely, as soon as the truck is moving, you can simply continue pushing it for quite some distance. Why is this? Physics. Your friends helped you break the inertia it takes to get the truck moving. Once it's moving, it's much easier to keep it moving. The weight hasn't changed, just your perception of it.

Lifting weights is the same. When a weight is too heavy for you to move in strict fashion, you'll start to cheat or bounce the weight to overcome inertia. That is exactly what doesn't make muscles grow.

Q. Seriously, where's the cardio?

A. We thought we covered this, but OK...there isn't any. Seriously, none. This program is about building muscle and nothing more. We're trying to achieve a certain result and cardio is going to inhibit that. If you MUST, and we mean absolutely must, do some cardio, one high-intensity interval training (HIIT) session a week is all that we'll allow, though we do encourage you to fight this urge as well. There will be time for that once you've got your hard-earned muscle. *Brett's Note:* I tried to sneak cardio in for the first few weeks and wasn't seeing the same results until I cut. It. Out. After completing the program, I focused on 3 sessions of HIIT a week and combined it with the Intermediate program.

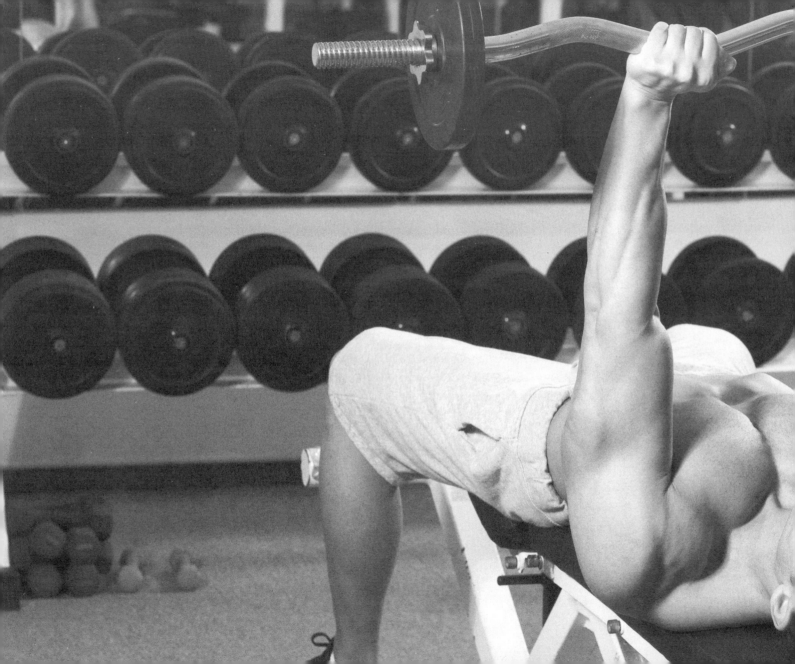

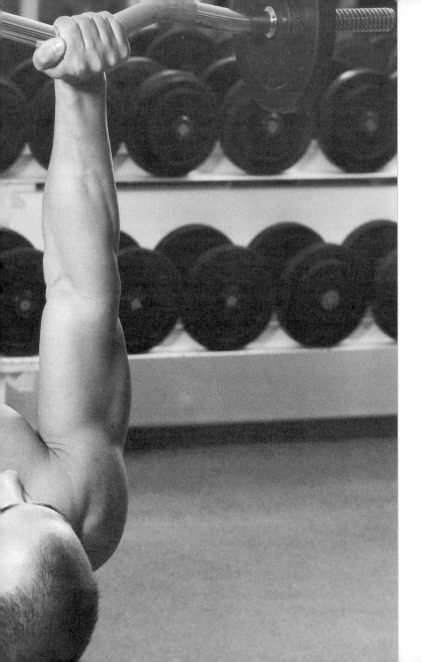

PART II:
WORKOUT
PROGRAMS

Before You Begin

Guess what? We're going to tell you to get off your ass and go to the doctor before you start this program. How does right now work for you?

BRETT: Let me guess: the last time you went to the doctor, Dylan was still a regular on *Beverly Hills 90210*, right? What is it about guys that make them afraid to go to the doctor for an annual checkup, especially when the doctor could help decode almost all of your aches and pains and give you some insight into how good a job you're doing taking care of the ol' bod? Chances are, you're a 20-minute visit away from a clean bill of health.

Even if they do find anything alarming, you're much better off to catch it early than have it sneak up on you later. My wife, Kristen, absolutely forbade me from training for Ironman Arizona in 2009 until after I received a doctor's sign-off, and I'm glad I did. Hundreds of hours running, biking and swimming would've been a foolish undertaking had I not had my ticker checked out first. Suck it up, make a call and go see your doc.

Here's the disclaimer: Always obtain clearance from a doctor that you are healthy enough to begin this or any other strenuous exercise regimen. Perform each exercise—especially heavy lifts—within your ability and always use available restraints, safety equipment and proper form. Most of all, don't be stupid and lift too much, too fast—that's a recipe for a pulled muscle or a bout of DOMS (delayed onset muscle soreness) that will knock you off-track from completing the next workout.

Now that we've got that little detail out of the way, before we start talking about the specific programs, we need to be clear again: This is a muscle-building program, not a strength program. There are massive programming differences between training for strength and training for muscle mass and size, also generally known as muscular hypertrophy. For instance, strength training is about finding advantages to lift more weights while hypertrophy training is solely focused on increasing muscle size and definition. When one trains for strength, the weight lifted is the only measure of success. Hypertrophy is concerned with muscle size, definition and symmetry and cares less about overall weight and more about the effects of the weight lifted.

We wanted to reiterate this not because strength has no place in training for muscle size; in fact, the opposite is true. Rather, we want to be clear about the goals of the program and the reason you're reading this book: to increase lean muscle mass.

And now that we've established where we're trying to go, we can talk about how we're going to get there. Over the years, many different training programs have been talked about as being "the best" for growing muscle. The simple truth is that all of these programs can and do work to some degree because overstimulating muscles will lead to growth. The problems start to emerge when you talk about optimizations for experience, time in the gym, time to achieve your goals and overcoming stagnation. Couple that with the fact that certain styles of training will be more beneficial for some than others and you end up with near religious fervor over training programs.

We take a different approach. Instead of choosing one side, we've combined the best of several divergent programs and styles to produce a workout program capable of achieving amazing results in minimal time for nearly every person working out in the gym today. The most advanced bodybuilders in the world might find flaws in this program, but if you aren't posing on stage in a thong somewhere, this program is likely more effective than whatever system you're using today.

7 Weeks to 10 Pounds of Muscle Program

In this chapter you'll find details on the three basic training styles and how our programs will use the best of each approach to produce the best muscle-building workouts possible. Learn about each method and their benefits and drawbacks, then jump into the programs.

Our programs are divided into Prep, Intermediate and Advanced. Each program is designed to achieve a specific result. We recommend everyone start in Prep and only move on to Intermediate when you've achieved certain strength numbers. The Advanced Program combines all the styles of training into one devilishly effective routine and, trust us on this, you won't want to start that until you've been through both Prep and Intermediate.

Training Styles

Each style of training has a base philosophy that can achieve decent results by itself, but combined they work even better. Understanding each style's strengths and weaknesses will allow you to understand when and where to use them effectively.

STRENGTH TRAINING

Strength: increasing base strength, fun program to follow, ego boosting

Weakness: increasing muscle size

Classic strength training is only concerned with increasing the amount of weight a person can lift. In powerlifting, this is achieved through body position, hand, foot and bar positions, not to mention those wicked-sweet man-i-tards some guys use to increase their lifting power. We won't be doing any of that, though we will incorporate exercises to increase core strength.

Strength has many advantages and should be the base of any good hypertrophy program. One of the failings of pure volume or tension programs is they do not incorporate a strength component. And while volume and tension training can be more effective at increasing muscle size than strength training alone, combined they achieve more than they could apart.

Our approach to strength training is called progressive overloading, meaning we'll continually strive to add more weight to the bar for a prescribed set of reps and sets. In practice, we want you to add weight each workout as long as you can continue to hit your reps and sets number. When you can no longer lift for the prescribed reps in a set, you hold steady until you can. This means you'll be taxing your muscles each and every workout in a progressive way, and you should be able to continually achieve new maximum lifts for quite some time. This approach is naturally immune to stagnation as you'll theoretically never be doing the same workout twice. Naturally there will be a time when you can't lift more; there is of course an upper limit to just how strong you can get! But don't worry—it will take quite some time before you find this ceiling. Bottom line: you'll always be trying to move up in weight for strength-training sets.

VOLUME TRAINING

Strength: increasing muscle size, great for combination lifts

Weakness: increasing muscle strength, need to check your ego

Volume training is primarily concerned with the overall volume, meaning number of reps and sets, per workout. To achieve a higher number of reps and sets, the overall weight of exercises needs to be reduced, sometimes by as much as 50%–70% depending on the muscle group being worked. Volume training is where you'll feel the "pump" that you might hear others talk about. What happens is the muscles get a rush of blood from all the activity and grow accordingly. Of course, this "pump" is only temporary, but the results of increasing the overall load on the muscle will be eventual growth.

An aspect of volume training that's often overlooked is the ego issue. You'll be lifting much lighter weights than you would for your 1-rep or 5-rep max, and you'll be using very strict form. You'll see others around the gym bouncing heavy weights and you'll be tempted to give in to your ego and start to increase the weights. This is a huge mistake and will only hurt you in the long run. Be sure of yourself and the approach, be consistent and you'll achieve more than those people bouncing heavy weights to be able to lift them. It's commonly said that when you bounce heavy weights, the only thing that grows is your ego.

Our approach to volume training is pretty classic. Volume training works well for most muscles, but it's best for the big movers. Legs, chest and shoulders all respond well to volume training. Smaller muscles achieve good results through volume training, but we have a better

approach for them later. For now we'll keep the volume for the bigger muscle groups.

Lastly, you won't move up in weight when volume training until you can do the prescribed number of reps and sets. That is the nature of volume training; the reps and sets are more important than the weight.

TENSION TRAINING

Strength: increasing muscle size and hardness, particularly in isolation exercises

Weakness: extremely taxing on the central nervous system, requires extreme mental fortitude

Classic tension training has two main components: time under tension and constant tension. Time under tension, or TUT, deals with the total time a muscle is worked, meaning the total number of seconds in a work set. Constant tension means keeping tension on the muscle for the entire work set, meaning you won't fully lock out a joint during a set.

Tension training programs typically incorporate either or both of these approaches. Our approach will blend them into one tension work set called Rest-Pause.

Rest-Pause is a tension style where for a certain lift you keep constant tension on the muscle being worked for the entire work set—you never fully lock out and you use a very slow and methodical movement. The movement should be slow: 5–8 seconds down, 1–2 seconds up. No bouncing of the weights, ever! You work the exercise to failure and then release the muscle tension by putting the weight down or racking it. Take 10–15 deep breaths and then go again for as many reps as you can, again putting the weight down when reaching failure. Take another 10–15 deep breaths and go once more until failure. That's considered 1 Rest-Pause set, and the total number of reps between the pauses is the total number for the Rest-Pause set. In practice, a typical Rest-Pause set might be 8 reps, 10-second pause, 4 reps, 10-second pause, 2 reps, for a total of 16 reps.

One progresses in a Rest-Pause set by meeting certain rep requirements for a certain weight. We say that once you achieve 15 reps at a certain weight, feel free to move up in weight for the next workout. However, if you fail to get 10 reps at the new weight, go back down to the previous weight until you reach 18 or 20 reps. That's how you bust through plateaus in Rest-Pause exercises.

As with volume training, you'll be using much less weight than you would for your 1-rep or 5-rep max. Resist the urge to cheat, bounce weight or decrease the time on the descent. This is the single most common mistake with both volume and tension training and it hurts overall progress in the long run.

Now that we've gone over the various training program styles we're going to jump into the nitty gritty of our approach. As stated earlier, nearly everyone reading this should go through the Prep Program regardless of how fit they think they are.

The programs are set up to build on each other. You'll notice that the Prep Program is incorporated into the Intermediate Program, which is also incorporated in the Advanced Program. This is intentional as (1) it builds confidence, (2) it actually sets you up for success by progressively adding instead of jumping and (3) you can see how a lifelong program can be formed and tweaked.

Reading the Charts

For each workout day, the chart indicates what lift you should do, as well as the number of reps and sets. To determine weight and intensity, the workout style is also given. *Warm-Up* means this is a warm-up set; you're using light weights and low reps to prepare your joints and muscles for more intensity. *Normal* means a normal bodybuilding set; you'll use relatively heavy weight for the indicated number of reps and sets. A *Drop Set* means you'll perform a single set of the same number of reps as the previous set using a lighter weight, usually 5–10 pounds less. The idea is to lower the weight so your fatigued muscles can complete all the reps. A *Power Set* means you're lifting the weight with explosive power: take 1 second to move the weight up, and 2–3 seconds to lower it back down. *Rest-Pause* means you'll do a single set to failure—that's as many reps as you can—then take 5 deep breaths, and go again. You'll do this three times total.

Prep Program

The Prep Program keeps it simple, focusing on strength training and just barely touching volume training. The purpose of this program is twofold. First, it's designed to get your body used to lifting weights, particularly heavier weights. Start to learn your body, know your limits and find out how your body reacts to the various lifts. This is also the time when you'll start to see how much weight you can handle for each lift. Second, the Prep Program will teach you to focus on form. You'll start the program using weights you can reasonably handle, and it is critically important you absolutely NAIL your form. As you progress to heavier weights, any slight mistakes in form could be disastrous, particularly with the big two: squats and deadlifts.

This program is slated for 4 weeks, though in reality it could be a lifelong workout program in and of itself. When you advance through the other programs in this book and reach the level of muscularity you want, you can use the Prep Program to maintain that level while still increasing strength. This is a great all-around program.

Testing Your Progress

If we were building a multi-year training program for someone, the Prep Program would serve not only as a gentle introduction, but it would also have exit criteria. You'd have to meet certain requirements in terms of how much weight you can lift to progress out of the program into the Intermediate stage. We can't be with you all the time when you work out, so there's no real requirement in place, but it is generally useful to know and understand what those are and why we would have such a requirement.

The strength requirements for passing onto the Intermediate Program are based on your body weight and the amount you can lift in your 1 rep maximum (1RM) on a particular exercise. They are as follows:

Squat (page 108)	1.5x your weight
Deadlift (page 111)	2x your weight
Bench Press	1.25x your weight
Overhead Press (page 112)	.75x your weight

So for example, here's how much you would have to lift if you weigh 150 or 200 pounds:

Your weight	Squat 1.5x	Deadlift 2x	Bench Press 1.25x	Overhead Press (page 112) .75x
200lb	300lb	400lb	250lb	150lb
150lb	225lb	300lb	187.5lb	112.5lb

These are by no means absolute maximums; you'll obviously be getting much stronger over time. These rough numbers mean you have achieved a certain level of strength that will greatly benefit you as the programs progress. It also means your body is sufficiently strong to protect itself as you add more volume and tension when you move into the Intermediate Program.

As you can see, these goals are not unreasonable, though chances are that you'll be less strong on one or two of the lifts than you would like. Those are your focus areas!

QUICK LIST OF STYLES AND ABBREVIATIONS *For further explanations of the workout styles, see pages 43–45.*	
Warm-Up	Warm-up set
Normal	Normal body-building set
Drop Set	Single drop after previous set
Power	Explosive power—1 second up, 2–3 seconds down
Rest-Pause	Single set to failure, then 5 deep breaths. Repeat 3 times.
AMAN / AMAP	As many as needed/possible. Complete as many reps as possible with good form.

Prep Program

Monday Bench Press

EXERCISE	STYLE	SETS	REPS	ALTERNATE
Flat Bench Press (page 114)	Warm-Up	3	10-20	
Flat Bench Press (page 114)	Normal	5	5	
Flat Bench Press (page 114)	Volume	3	12-20	

Tuesday Deadlift

Deadlift (page 111)	Warm-Up	AMAN	5	
Deadlift (page 111)	Reverse Pyramid	5	3,3,5,5,5	

Wednesday Rest

Thursday Overhead Press

Overhead Press (page 112)	Warm-Up	3	10	Dumbbell Press (page 113)
Overhead Press (page 112)	Normal	5	5	Dumbbell Press (page 113)
Overhead Press (page 112)	Volume	3	15-20	Dumbbell/Barbell Push Press (pages 112-13)

Prep Program

Friday Squat

	EXERCISE	STYLE	SETS	REPS	ALTERNATE
	Body Squat (page 109)	Warm-Up	3	12–15	
	Squat (page 108)	Warm-Up	AMAN	5	
	Squat (page 108)	Reverse Pyramid	5	3,3,5,5,5	Box Squat (page 109)
	Squat (page 108)	Volume	3	12–20	Box Squat (page 109) or Leg Press (page 120)

Saturday Rest

Sunday Rest

Intermediate Program

The Intermediate Program adds a major portion of volume training to the Prep Program and will start to feel very much like you are bodybuilding. By now you should have achieved certain strength numbers and you should continue to see those numbers rise as you move through the program. Now the focus is on actually increasing muscle size by adding a healthy dose of volume.

The Intermediate Program is a 4-week program designed to make you familiar with a bodybuilding-style workout, to continue to increase your strength and to pack on some good, quality muscle mass. Focus on reining in your ego and understanding your volume numbers. You'll be using much lighter weights than your 1RM and at first this can be disconcerting, particularly if others in the gym are putting up much higher weights, even if they're using poor form or training for different goals. Do not get caught up in this! Focus on yourself, your goals and learning as much about you, your body and your program as you can.

The actual weights you'll use will probably start around 50%–60% of your 1RM, maybe even lower. It is much more important that you hit the reps and sets than you use heavier weights in this part of the program. Again, the hardest part of this is going to be checking your ego and using the appropriate weight.

QUICK LIST OF STYLES AND ABBREVIATIONS	
For further explanations of the workout styles, see pages 43–45.	
Warm-Up	Warm-up set
Normal	Normal body-building set
Drop Set	Single drop after previous set
Power	Explosive power—1 second up, 2–3 seconds down
Rest-Pause	Single set to failure, then 5 deep breaths. Repeat 3 times.
AMAN / AMAP	As many as needed/possible. Complete as many reps as possible with good form.

Intermediate Program

Monday Chest (Major), Shoulders (minor), Triceps (minor)

EXERCISE	STYLE	SETS	REPS	ALTERNATE
Flat Bench Press (page 114)	Warm-Up	3	10–20	
Flat Bench Press (page 114)	Normal	5	5	
Flat Bench Press (page 114)	Volume	5	12–20	
Dumbbell Press (page 113)	Volume	5	12–20	Overhead Press (page 112)
Dip (page 118)	Normal	5	AMAP	

Tuesday Back (Major), Quadriceps (minor), Biceps (minor)

Deadlift (page 111)	Warm-Up	AMAN	5	
Deadlift (page 111)	Reverse Pyramid	5	3,3,5,5,5	
Leg Press (page 120)	Volume	3	15–20	Front Squat (page 110)
Barbell Row (page 122)	Normal	3	8	Low Bar Row (page 123) or 1-Arm Row (page 128)
Dumbbell Shrug (page 124)	Normal	3	8–10	Barbell Shrug (page 125)
EZ Bar Curl (page 126)	Normal	3	8–10	Hammer Curl (page 127)

Wednesday Core, Gluteus maximus

Weighted Hip Thrust (page 135)	Normal	2	10	
Bird Dog (page 138)	Normal	2	20 per side	
Plank (page 139)	Normal	2	1 minute	
optional: Landmine (page 136)	Normal	2	10 per side	
optional: Wood Chop (page 140)	Normal	2	3	Hammer Curl (page 127)

Intermediate Program

Thursday Shoulders (major), Chest (minor), Triceps (Minor)

EXERCISE	STYLE	SETS	REPS	ALTERNATE
Overhead Press (page 112)	Warm-Up	3	10	Dumbbell Press (page 113)
Overhead Press (page 112)	Normal	3	5	Dumbbell Press (page 113)
Overhead Press (page 112)	Volume	5	15–20	Dumbbell Push Press (page 113)
Dumbbell Bench Press	Normal	3	8–12	Flat Bench Press (page 114)
Close-Grip Bench Press (page 129)	Normal	3	8–10	Reverse-Grip Bench Press (page 114)
Shoulder Raise (page 130)	Rest-Pause	1	12–15	

Friday Legs (Major)

Body Squat (page 109)	Warm-Up	3	12–15	
Squat (page 108)	Warm-Up	AMAN	5	
Squat (page 108)	Reverse Pyramid	5	3,3,5,5,5	Box Squat (page 109)
Leg Press (page 120)	Volume	3	12–20	
Romanian Deadlift (page 133)	Normal	3	8–12	
Hamstring Curl (page 121)	Normal	5	8–12	
Calf Raise (page 132)	Normal	3	15	

Saturday Rest

Sunday Rest

Advanced Program

The Advanced Program pulls everything together with strength, volume and tension training. Incorporating all three training styles will tax even the most advanced weight lifters and you should only attempt this when you (1) have a good sense of your body and how it responds to weight, (2) have enough discipline and mental fortitude to see it through and (3) have your diet NAILED.

You'll be blasting your body and you'll need to feed it appropriately to help it recover and grow. This program is not for the faint of heart or mind. You should be prepared to work.

The main addition in the Advanced Program is the tension style of training with Rest-Pause sets (page 45). As with volume training, you'll be using much lower weights than your 1RM and you'll need to check your ego to achieve this.

QUICK LIST OF STYLES AND ABBREVIATIONS	
For further explanations of the workout styles, see pages 43–45.	
Warm-Up	Warm-up set
Normal	Normal body-building set
Drop Set	Single drop after previous set
Power	Explosive power—1 second up, 2–3 seconds down
Rest-Pause	Single set to failure, then 5 deep breaths. Repeat 3 times.
AMAN / AMAP	As many as needed/possible. Complete as many reps as possible with good form.

Advanced Program

Monday — Chest (Major), Shoulders (minor), Triceps (minor)

EXERCISE	STYLE	SETS	REPS	ALTERNATE
Flat Bench Press (page 114)	Warm-Up	3	10–20	
Flat Bench Press (page 114)	Normal	5	5	
Flat Bench Press (page 114)	Volume	5	12–20	
Overhead Press (page 112)	Volume	5	12–20	Overhead Press (page 112)
Incline Dumbbell Bench Press (page 116)	Rest-Pause	1	12–20	Incline Bench Press (page 116)
Dip (page 118)	Rest-Pause	1	12–15	
Triceps Pressdown (page 119)	Rest-Pause	1	12–15	

Tuesday — Back (Major), Quadriceps (minor), Biceps (minor)

EXERCISE	STYLE	SETS	REPS	ALTERNATE
Deadlift (page 111)	Warm-Up	AMAN	5	
Deadlift (page 111)	Reverse Pyramid	5	3,3,5,5,5	
Leg Press (page 120)	Volume	3	15–20	Front Squat (page 110)
Barbell Row (page 122)	Normal	3	8	
1-Arm Dumbbell Row (page 128)	Volume	3	12–20	
Dumbbell Shrug (page 124)	Rest-Pause	1	12–15	Barbell Shrug (page 125)
EZ Bar Curl (page 126)	Rest-Pause	1	12–15	Hammer Curl (page 127)

Wednesday — Core, Gluteus maximus

EXERCISE	STYLE	SETS	REPS	ALTERNATE
Weighted Hip Thrust (page 135)	Normal	2	10	
Bird Dog (page 138)	Normal	2	20 per side	
Plank (page 139)	Normal	2	1 minute	
optional: Landmine (page 136)	Normal	2	10 per side	
optional: Wood Chop (page 140)	Normal	2	5–8	

Advanced Program

Thursday Shoulders (major), Chest (minor), Triceps (Minor)

EXERCISE	STYLE	SETS	REPS	ALTERNATE
Overhead Press (page 112)	Warm-Up	3	10	Dumbbell Press (page 113)
Overhead Press (page 112)	Normal	3	5	Dumbbell Press (page 113)
Overhead Press (page 112)	Volume	5	15-20	Barbell/Dumbbell Push Press (pages 112-13)
Dumbbell Bench Press (page 114)	Volume	5	15-20	Flat Bench Press (page 114)
Dip (page 118)	Normal	3	AMAP	
Close-Grip Bench Press (page 129)	Rest-Pause	1	12-15	
Shoulder Raise (page 130)	Rest-Pause	1	12-15	

Friday Legs (Major)

EXERCISE	STYLE	SETS	REPS	ALTERNATE
Body Squat (page 109)	Warm-Up	3	12-15	
Squat (page 108)	Warm-Up	AMAN	5	
Squat (page 108)	Reverse Pyramid	5	3,3,5,5,5	Box Squat (page 109)
Leg Press (page 120)	Volume	3	12-20	
Romanian Deadlift (page 133)	Normal	3	8-12	
Hamstring Curl (page 121)	Volume	5	12-20	
Calf Raise (page 132)	Rest-Pause	1	12-15	

Saturday Rest

Sunday Rest

Reflections on the Programs

JASON: I love this hypertrophy workout, and with good reason. This workout, coupled with the diet outlined in Part III, helped me gain 20 pounds of muscle in just over three months.* Frankly, I'm in love with this. But I had to work for it. There were times when I wanted to take the easy way out of the workout, but I knew if I did that I would only be cheating myself.

* What? Three months? Isn't this program only 7 weeks? We spent months testing out many different programs—some positive, some negative—before we nailed this one down. While writing this book, I've tested, trained, learned and grown quite a bit!

I'll admit, though, that there were days when I wasn't feeling up for another set of squats, so I moved to the leg press. However, I pushed myself on the leg press! I was already "cheating" myself a bit; no way was I going to waste my time! And in the end, that is what this is all about, right? Maximizing our time in the gym to achieve our goals?

More importantly, and this is personal, I learned things about myself and what works best for my body that I can take with me for the rest of my life. I learned that my biceps do not respond to heavy curls, mostly because I cheat them too much. Instead, I can get great biceps results from tension volume training and Rest-Pause-style training. I learned that my squats are king, and if I want to get big, strong legs I need to squat, not hack squat or leg press. I learned that I can't engage my lats unless I focus very intently.

And I also learned that I can let my ego get the best of me and start to stray from the plan. Stick with the plan, focus on yourself and don't think about the weights others are using.

What I Did Right: Early on I focused very well on strength training. My numbers on lifts went up with each workout and I began to get addicted to seeing those numbers increase. It was extremely motivating. I also learned quite a bit about how my body responds to certain lifts and certain styles. I found that I responded to squats much better than I did to leg press. I also found that I prefer low-bar squats to high-bar squats.

I also played with foot and hand placement on all my lifts and found the combinations that made me the most comfortable and still engaged the muscles the most. This will be highly individual, and do not let anyone tell you that any one hand or foot placement is universal. You decide based on your body and how it responds.

What I Did Wrong: I got addicted to seeing my strength numbers go up and focused too much on strength at the expense of volume. There was a small window of time where I got much stronger but not much bigger. I regret not focusing more on volume and tension during this window of time as I feel I could have achieved even more size!

I also didn't check my ego early enough, particularly with tension training. You won't start to feel the tension until later in the set, maybe as late as the sixth or tenth rep. It was a mistake to use too heavy a weight to begin with. I should have used less weight and focused on feeling the tension and going slower, engaging more muscle fibers.

BRETT: I already covered ad nauseam the fact that this program was way out of my comfort zone, right? Well, only a few weeks or so into the required intense lifting I had a few awesome breakthroughs:

1. I deadlifted more than double my body weight. Actually, pretty easily. Never in my wildest dreams did I imagine that I'd be able to deadlift over 355 pounds. Never.

2. After some testing, I found the right foods and timing to maximize my muscle gain, and it quickly became second nature.

3. I felt solid. Size medium shirts started to stretch a little tighter across chest and my arms actually filled the sleeves; I started to see the exact results I was looking for even more quickly than I had expected.

4. After a couple weeks of puffiness due to the increase in carbs while I was modifying my diet, my six-pack abs came back.

Number 3 was really the goal I wanted to achieve for my own physique the first time through the program, but I was also very cognizant of keeping my abs visible. I had put a lot of effort into making steady progress to keep my core well-defined since the initial 7 Weeks to 50 Pull-Ups photo shoot and was initially bummed as I lost definition while modifying my daily nutrition. Jason kept reassuring me that if I stuck with the plan I'd get my defined abs back before the seven weeks were complete, and I was thrilled to see the results of muscle gain while also welcoming back my abs.

What I Did Right: I made up my mind on day one that I was going to take at least two months off from marathon and triathlon training and put 100% effort into this program. Truth be told, I "cheated" a little bit and continued playing soccer two nights a week and ran a few obstacle races and a couple 10Ks. In my defense, I did cut my daily mileage down to nearly zero and didn't spend any time on the treadmill.

The biggest thing I did right was sticking with the routine and getting results. I spent some time testing out the different nutritional protocols to find the timing and amounts that worked for me.

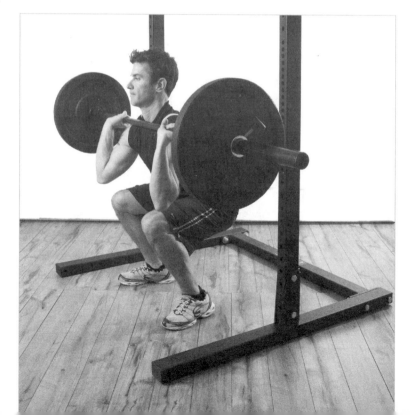

What I Did Wrong: Early on, I was eating poorly and my meal timing was way off. By poorly, I mean I was stuck in my old ways of eating more protein than carbs and not fueling well after a hard training session. Eating more calories than I was used to was a little tough to get used to, and a bit hard on my stomach. Make no mistake; if you stop eating, you will stop growing! After about 10 days of not taking in enough of the right calories at the right time, I felt like I was spinning my wheels. Luckily, I only had to refocus on how I was fueling to get back on track.

As I mentioned on page 30, workout ADD can screw up any plan—and, yes, I am very guilty! It's not that I had trouble sticking to the lifting plan, but I kept adding extra exercises into the mix during workouts and even going to the park each morning for dips, pull-ups, push-ups and core work. I was sabotaging my results by overtraining the same muscles each day. This actually lowers your body's ability to produce testosterone and for the muscle fibers to heal and grow. Oops.

Last but not least, I was extremely afraid of losing endurance by not running 25-plus miles a week and fretted about this for nearly the entire program. My fears were unfounded. When I finished up the program I hosted a 13.1-mile trail run with some friends in North Phoenix and we had a blast. My only issue was some lingering pain from a sprained ankle from soccer (but that's a totally different story). My endurance was just fine; definitely not at peak levels when I train 50-plus miles a week, but my running speed and distance came back very quickly, and my new-found muscle didn't weigh me down. Instead, it gave me additional power to push through tough terrain and surely made me feel more stable on rocky, rugged trails.

What I've Learned: One of the interesting things about being a guinea pig for all the programs in the 7 Weeks series and being in the photos you see in each of the books is that my physique is a work in progress. If you don't believe that, just look at my photos from back when I started the 7 Weeks books and where I am now. I received an e-mail from one of the nearly 20,000 registered members of www.7weekstofitness.com that asked me who the "older guy" (me) was in *7 Weeks to 50 Pull-Ups*:

"I have a confession make. I actually made fun of you in the pictures in the pull-up book. I said to myself, why would they put this older guy in this book? He's not like the guy on the cover! Then when I found out who you were and then your other books came out and before my eyes how you transformed your body to what it is today. I get it now...after I put my foot in my mouth! I realized you were the perfect guinea pig for this system to prove that it works, it really works, and you are living proof! You showed that anybody can transform their body if they want to. I apologize for judging a book by its cover. If it wasn't for your heart and determination, everybody you've helped with these books wouldn't have taken the challenge that changed our lives. Brett, you inspire and you're the man! Thanks again!" —Sean Sullivan

I've since talked to Sean many times, and have thanked him for what I consider to be an amazing compliment. I'm really happy that he understood what Jason and I are doing and how we hope to help others change their lives.

My personal journey is not about seven weeks, gaining 10 pounds of muscle, getting ripped, doing a ridiculous amount of pull-ups, sit-ups or any other short-term accomplishments. My health and fitness goals are much longer-term. As a kid, I was awkward and pudgy. As a teen I was a little less awkward (or so I thought, the photos tend to prove otherwise) but was never fit. In my 20s my weight ballooned and I started smoking pretty heavily and really let myself go. I was as unhappy with my life choices as I was with my fitness and physique. Throughout my 30s I scrambled to figure it out, and by 35 I was on the right track. Right around the time I was turning 40, I nailed it and saw all the years of toiling start to pay off. My partnership with Jason in bringing you all these fitness books blossomed at the same time, and continues to expand. These books, exercises, programs and nutritional guidelines are an homage to years of hard work, research, failed attempts to get fit, nutritional mistakes, injuries caused by improper form, overtraining

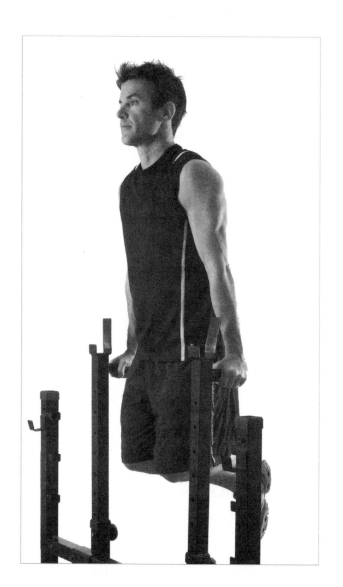

or our own stupidity and all the sweet successes of setting a new marathon personal best, finishing my first Ironman, becoming a fitness model with an actual six-pack (probably the most unlikely outcome of all) and being so happy in my own skin and healthy, enjoying life with my family and friends, participating in events with my kids and watching them blossom, sharing every day with the love of my life, Kristen, who made it all possible.

She saw something in me that I failed to recognize; inside there was a better man than the overweight smoker she met in 2000. It took a while for me to realize some of my potential, and without her support it would never have been possible.

Keep in mind that Jason's and my results are not necessarily the same as yours—we sincerely hope you do even better!

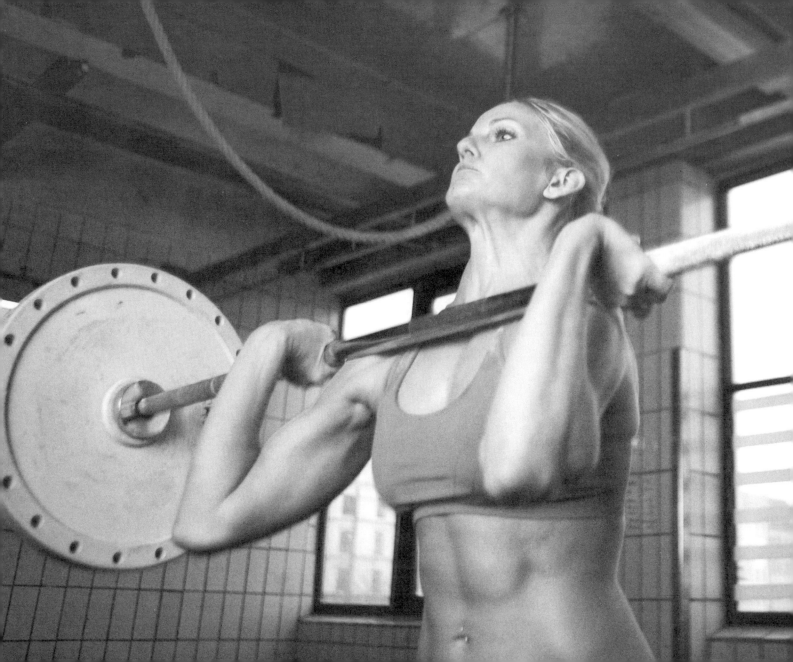

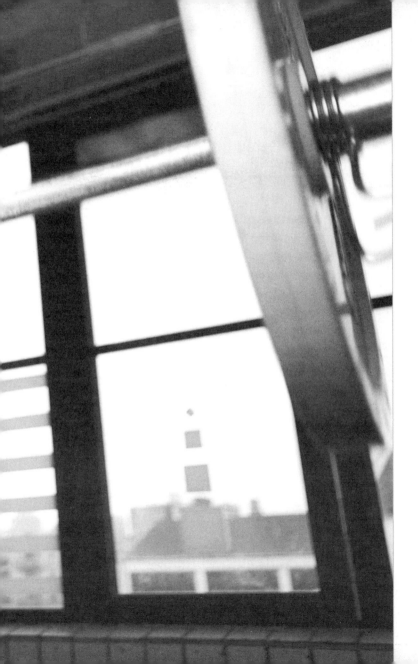

PART III:
NUTRITION
PROGRAM

Eat More, Gain More

Quick quiz: What's this book about? Gaining muscle, nothing more. We are about to talk about nutrition that packs on muscle, fuels your workouts and generally supports achieving the singular goal of gaining muscle. This is NOT a general nutrition program. We in no way advocate you follow what we outline below for the rest of your life or for general fitness. Instead, we're going to talk about eating to grow and gain muscle for a specific period of time while following a specific regimen.

BRETT: While I follow the "extreme" version of the nutritional program only when I'm focusing on muscle gain, throughout the year I will use the "Safe" and "Basic" versions quite a bit based on my level of training and goals. The bottom line is you need to pick a nutritional program that matches your specific goals and not just stick with the same one year-round. Match your workouts with the proper nutrition.

Our Nutrition Philosophy

We wanted to title this section "Everything Old Is New Again" because, frankly, most of what we're going to lay out is stuff we've known in one form or another for years or even decades. That's not to say that there has ever been as comprehensive a program for gaining muscle as this; there hasn't. We've put together all the information in one easy-to-use guide that anyone can follow. And while we might have "known" many of the whats, we didn't know many of the whys. That's the difference between 1973 and 2013. Essentially, we've brought together the science, trends, information and "bro-science" and gotten rid of the garbage advice to give you only the best of what works. Nothing more, nothing less. If you want to know how to grow muscle, this is the place to be.

And so we'll jump right in and begin by laying out our food philosophy: Bottom line, nothing is off limits. This program is extremely laid-back about what exact foods to eat. It's all good so long as it is used to support the goal of gaining muscle. One caveat: It's up to you to do a little bit of show and tell in the mirror each day to figure out what works best for you (we'll touch on that a bit later). Last, too much of a bad thing is still a bad thing; avoid loading up on excessive sugar, salt, any trans fat, preservatives and chemicals like aspartame.

That being said, we have some awesome recipes for the foodies out there that were created by our incredibly skilled chef, Corey Irwin. Get ready to put some inspiration into your meals. Browse Corey's recipes starting on page 93.

More important than the specific foods you eat is when you eat them. Many diets out there talk about calories and/or percentage of nutrients but do little to tell you when to eat that food. Over the past few years, more and more evidence has also shown that the timing of food is equally important, if not more than, the amount you eat.

And to that end, we won't ever ask you to count calories. That's right, no counting calories, honestly. Calories historically offered an easy and convenient, yet imperfect, understanding of how food impacts our body. Much like our overall understanding of the complex machine that is the body, our understanding of weight loss, maintenance and growth have changed. That isn't to say the fundamentals aren't the same, just that we understand that calories are rather simplistic and don't tell the whole story. Even so, calories offer a common, convenient language. We'll still talk about "overall caloric intake" as an easy way to say "eat more!" We won't be throwing out the caloric baby with the bathwater!

Instead of counting calories, we'll talk about macros and timing: protein, fat and carbohydrates, how many you need per day and when you need them. With this in mind, we can begin to talk about what it takes to grow muscle.

Eating to Grow Muscle

If you want to sculpt your physique and pack on the muscle, you must first start in the kitchen. Eating right is 80 percent of the battle. Sure, you've got to strength train to get and stay buff, which is the other very crucial 20 percent, but you've also got to actively pay attention to what you're putting into your mouth and stay in control of your choices. After all, you and you alone are responsible for deciding what you eat. The keys to success in this regard are simple: Remain aware of your food intake and plan out your meals in advance. To that end, we have tips to help you accomplish both.

In order to pack on 10 pounds of lean muscle, you'll need to change two major aspects of your eating. First, up your total weekly caloric intake by increasing your three macros: fat, protein and carbs. The second thing you'll need to change, and by far the most important, is the amount and timing of those macros. If that sounds confusing, don't fret. You've got a secret weapon from a very unlikely source: carbs.

Secret Weapon

Want to gain muscle? Want to get bigger? Want to dramatically change your appearance? There are two things you need in your arsenal: heavy weights and carbohydrates. We've already talked about the heavy weights, so now we'll turn to the carbs.

Carbs, specifically carb timing, is the single most important thing to nailing in your diet as you fight to gain muscle.

The second old-school secret to carbs is carb cycling: alternating days of high and low carbs depending on your activity level. This is a classic bodybuilding technique to gain lean muscle while keeping fat gain to an absolute minimum. This old method has been revamped in many modern approaches, and we'll share what we've found to be the most effective.

Carbs—The Most Misunderstood Macronutrient

Before we get into the actual principles and structure of the diet, we want to address some common myths and rumors about carbs.

First, carbohydrates are just molecules the body uses as its primary source of energy. Carbohydrates are turned into glucose, the form of sugar transported and used by the body. In fact, carbs are more readily converted to glucose than either fat or protein, meaning the body would prefer carbs to fat and protein when given the choice. Simple carbs, such as sugar, honey, jam, and most fruit drinks and soft drinks are sugars that are easily absorbed into the bloodstream. Complex carbs are those found in green vegetables, whole-grain breads, oatmeal and beans, as well as starchy vegetables such as potatoes, sweet corn and pumpkin. Since complex carbs are found in whole foods, they are also excellent sources for other vitamins and minerals and make up part of a healthy diet.

Which is all to say that carbs are not evil. There is nothing intrinsically wrong with them. Rather, "carb abuse" or loading up on low-quality carbs morning, noon and night is the real problem. Not understanding how carb intake affects your body and its hormonal patterns has led to an-all out attack on carbs in modern society, and for good reason. Carbs are the only macronutrient that is not needed by the body—at all. Fats and protein are essential macronutrients, meaning your body needs them to survive. Not so for carbs. A person could survive and never eat a crumb of bread or a bite of apple in their life. And that fact has led some to believe that carbs are evil, and in the common case, we tend to agree.

A shallow look at our society and the trend toward obesity, as well as our burgeoning understanding of how carbohydrates affect our bodies, has led health-conscious people to eat fewer carbs. And we actively invite people who are heading toward obesity to limit their carbs because, frankly, they should. Not only are they not priming their body to use carbs, but carbs will only get in the way of their real goal: weight loss. Even the general public, the ones who might not be obese (yet) but aren't overly active should also limit their carbs because they simply aren't active enough to properly use those nutrients in an effective way. Rather, an overconsumption of carbs will over time lead to weight gain and, if unchecked, obesity.

But this book isn't for those people. Carbohydrates are essential to the goal of gaining muscle. The advice in this book is for people willing to put in the work to do things differently and to make a huge change in their lives.

Carbs and Goals

Carbs are an interesting macronutrient, and depending on your goal, your usage of carbs will vary widely. By definition, if you are reading this book, you are looking to put on solid muscle and we'll need those carbs to do that.

This book, the eating programs we lay out and specifically the carb intake we suggest are NOT for the general public, are not for people unwilling to lift heavy weights and are not for those looking to shed some unwanted body fat. If your goal is to gain muscle and you are willing to put in the time and work by lifting heavy weights, by all means, read on. However, if the idea of lifting heavy weights scares you or if you are mostly interested in losing weight, we suggest you stop reading here and pick up a different book in our series, *7 Weeks to Getting Ripped*.

Basic Nutrition Principles

At this point we've established our goals and talked about the necessity of lifting heavy weights. But lifting alone won't cut it! If all we did were lift heavy weights, we would have essentially primed the body for growth but wouldn't be fueling that growth without changing our diet. So with that, we need to talk about our basic food and eating principles.

These principles are the basis for the programs laid out later in the chapter. Understanding the principles will allow you to adjust and adapt the programs to suit your needs and individual body.

1. SKIP BREAKFAST.

For the purpose of gaining solid muscle, breakfast can actually have detrimental effects on reshaping your body by cutting into the morning high-fat-burning window and priming your body for fat storage. If you must eat breakfast, a high-protein, zero-carb, moderate/low-fat breakfast is best. We don't recommend breakfast to anyone except the hardest of gainers and, frankly, even they should skip it.

Why? When you wake up, your body is at the highest point of insulin sensitivity for the entire day. If you did nothing different during the day, your body would slowly become more insulin insensitive as the day progresses. Eating food, specifically carbs, and to a lesser degree fat, when you are insulin sensitive is a great way to gain fat— that's not the goal we're shooting for!

2. THE LATER IN THE DAY YOU WORK OUT, THE BETTER.

We've found this to be the hardest to implement in practice, but it has the most upside. The later in the day you work out, the more food options you have and the better your gains will be. The optimal time to work out would be any time after 4 p.m. (assuming normal sleeping patterns). Due to your schedule, there will be times when you need to work out at noon and thereby have fewer food options later in the day. If you can work out later in the day, you can get away with eating more fun foods than you can earlier in the day.

Why? As we said in our advice that you skip breakfast, as the day progresses your body becomes less sensitive to insulin spikes, meaning it becomes harder to store food as fat. Working out later in the day primes the body to build muscle. And by fueling with carbs and protein, your body will be packing on solid slabs of muscle and minimal or no fat.

3. PROTEIN AND FAT ONLY BEFORE A WORKOUT.

Assuming for the sake of argument you work out after 5 p.m., eat only protein and fat before your workout and limit the total caloric intake to roughly 30 percent of your total for the day. This might be rough for some people, but you want to save your calories for when your body is going to use them the most: post-workout. The reason to only eat protein and fat and not carbs is that you have not primed your body to use the carbs yet; you haven't worked out.

Why? Special things happen when you lift heavy weights, but before you lift, you can't take advantage of them. In essence, the body is not ready to take use carbs well, and by eating carbs when the body is not ready makes it much more likely those carbs will be stored as fat, not muscle. So before a workout, it's best to fuel your body with fats and proteins.

4. PROTEIN AND CARBS ONLY AFTER A WORKOUT.

Immediately after your hard and heavy workout, your body is ready to grow. You've stimulated your body and put it in a position to soak up nutrients and repair muscle fibers. Now is the time to feed it! Eat protein to help the muscles repair and grow and carbs to shuttle the protein to the muscle. It's as simple as that.

5. NO WORKOUT? NO CARBS.

This is an easy rule to follow and you can immediately see the application. If you don't work out very hard with heavy weights, don't even think about eating carbs. Non-workout days? Fats and protein, baby!

Why? We can't state this enough. Carbs are only for post-workout when you've primed your body to grow. If you haven't worked out yet, or you are on a rest day, you haven't stressed your body; therefore, it can't and won't use the carbs to grow muscle. So why would you give it carbs? If you wanted to gain fat, non-workout days would be a perfect time to eat carbs, but that isn't our goal.

6. FOOD TYPE IS OVERRATED.

Clean foods, organic sources, grass-fed, non-farmed, etc. It gets confusing and, we're happy to say, is completely overrated. It is far more important to nail your macro levels and the timing of the food rather than the type of food. We have a saying: "First optimize what food you eat, then optimize what food your food eats."

The one and only caveat to the above is the type of carb. There is one time during the day the type of carb matters: Post-workout you want high-GI carbs (think dextrose, white rice and white potato). The sooner you spike your insulin and get your body rebuilding muscle, the better. Our recommended post-workout shake has whey protein isolate, creatine, leucine and dextrose—all the things a growing body needs!

7. KEEP AN EATING WINDOW.

One of the early mistakes Jason made was having too big a carb window, meaning he worked out too early in the day and freely ate carbs until he went to sleep. There are two ways to keep a window: work out later in the day so your natural window is between your workout and bed, or to still work out earlier, say noon, and eat your carbs for only a two-hour or so window. The approach you take is up to you. You will need to watch how you react and adjust accordingly. We strongly recommend you work out later in the day to have a natural window between the workout and going to bed.

The Science behind It All

Big caveat here: If you don't care about the why, you can more than safely skip this chapter. We strive to be practical in our advice, but we felt it was important to make sure we explained why we've made some rather radical recommendations. Again, if you don't care, move along!

Another caveat: The science here is piecemeal. There is no one authoritative study done that has drawn all these conclusions. Rather, many different people, institutions and studies have made portions of these conclusions based on recent findings. Most of what is found supports what bodybuilders and athletes have "known" and done for years. If you have done much Internet research into bodybuilding or gaining muscle, you've surely come across elements of what we suggest in various forms. As is the nature of research, we all stand on shoulders of others and advance the knowledge. We are no different. We thank everyone who puts in the time and energy to advance our collective knowledge and are quite happy to offer our own humble contribution.

Insulin

Insulin is the hormone that signals the body to grow, and it's the body's most anabolic hormone, meaning that it promotes growth nearly indiscriminately. In an overly simplified nutshell, insulin shuttles nutrients around your body into your muscles, liver and fat. So what if there was a way to pick and choose where the body stored the nutrients you fed it?

There is. Insulin sensitivity is highest when you wake up in the morning, and it goes down as the day progresses. This means that later in the day, your body won't react as strongly to the insulin release that results when you eat insulin-spiking foods, better known as carbohydrates. This is why we say that the morning isn't

a great time to be eating carbs: It would lead to fat gain, unless you prime the body to use the insulin spike for muscle growth.

The truth is that later in the day, both fat and muscle growth are lower. But training with heavy weights changes the dynamic and gives you the ability to control how your body uses insulin and where it stores it. Lifting heavy weights alters how your body will react to a spike in insulin and basically turns your muscles into sponges waiting to soak up nutrients. After a lifting workout, your muscle cells are more sensitive to insulin for an extended period of time (some research says up to 48 hours). This means that when you work out later in the day, during your post-training window, only your muscles—and not your fat—are ready to actually use the carbs you eat and use the resulting insulin spike to grow.

All this leads to the conclusion that for maximum muscle growth without an increase in fat, you need to work out at night and follow that workout with copious amounts of carbs, particularly high-GI carbs like white bread, rice and potatoes. High-GI carbs are broken down in the body more quickly than low-GI carbs are, meaning they will be out of your bloodstream before they can be stored as fat.

Macro Breakdown

When it comes to how much food a person should eat, there is just no simple answer. If you think of it like a formula for which you need to start satisfying certain requirements, then things usually fall into place.

The key will be paying attention to your body and how it reacts to your nutrition and exercise day in and day out. Once you are in tune with the day to day, small adjustments become trivial and you are able to make very good controlled gains.

When it comes to the three macronutrients—protein, fat and carbs—we start with protein. Shoot for 1 gram per pound of bodyweight you want to weigh. This number stays constant on workout and non-workout days. On non-workout days, protein should be roughly 50% of your macro breakdown and fat should be the rest. On workout days, protein should still be roughly 50%, but approximately 70% of your total calories should come AFTER your workout, meaning they should have a healthy dose of carbs. That being the case, it is going to be up to you to figure out how many grams of carbs and fat you will need. Quick summary so far:

The table might look intimidating at first, but it is really quite simple in practice. It will take time for you to acclimate your thinking to this, but once you do, it becomes second nature.

And when it becomes second nature you can start to muck around with the macros and adjust to your needs. The two main adjustments would be to up the overall calorie level on workout days and to start adding more carbs to the post-workout window. As far as overall calorie level, you should be at a slight deficit on non-workout days and a surplus on workout days. As you see how you are gaining (or not), you can start making your adjustments.

And remember: No one can tell you exactly how many grams of carbs, protein and fat to eat a day to get to where you want to be. It simply isn't possible because your body is individual and will react differently than everyone else's. The basics are the same, but the specifics need tweaking for you as an individual. It is far more important that you understand the principles so you can make the adjustments needed for you as an individual.

	PROTEIN (% of total calories)	FAT (% of total calories)	CARBS (% of total calories)
Workout Day: Pre-workout	15%	15%	0%*
Workout Day: Post-workout	25–35%	0%	35–45%
Non-Workout Day	50%	50%	0%*

* Keeping carbs at zero is more a mindset than a hard and fast rule. As long as you stay under 30 grams, you'll be fine.

The 7-Week Muscle-Building Nutrition Plan

Now, onto the program! We'll begin by offering what you might eat on a typical workout day, give options for what time you exercise and give a sample off day. Then we'll dive into details. When you have a firm understanding of why we have laid out the program as it is, feel free to tweak the program. Later in this chapter we give examples of how to manipulate the program based on your needs. But until you know how your body is going to respond, we recommend you stick with the basic program as it is laid out.

Basic Program

Essentially, the program works like this: After workouts, eat foods that are high in protein and carbs, and low in fat. On non-workout days, eat foods that are high in protein and fat, and low in carbs.

7-Week Muscle-Build Nutrition Plan

	NON-WORKOUT DAY (Typical)	WORKOUT DAY: 6:00 a.m. workout	WORKOUT DAY: Noon workout	WORKOUT DAY: 3:00 p.m. workout
6:00 a.m.	--	Workout	--	--
7:00 a.m.	Breakfast: none, black coffee	--	Breakfast: none, black coffee	Breakfast: none, black coffee
7:30 a.m.	--	Post-workout shake	--	--
Noon	--	Breakfast: none, black coffee	Workout	--
1:00 p.m.	Meal: protein + fat	Light meal: protein + carbs	--	Light meal: protein + fat
1:30 p.m.	--	--	Post-workout shake	--
3:00 p.m.	--	--	--	Workout
3:30 p.m.	--	Light meal: protein + carbs	Light meal: protein +carbs	--
4:30 p.m.	--	--	--	Post-workout shake
5:30 p.m.	Meal: protein + fat	Meal: protein + carbs	Meal: protein + carbs	Meal: protein + carbs
7:30 p.m.	Meal/snack: protein + fat	Meal/snack: protein + carbs	Meal/snack: protein + carbs	Meal/snack: protein + carbs
9:30 p.m.	--	Meal/snack: protein + carbs	Meal/snack: protein + carbs	Meal/snack: protein + carbs

PROGRAM NOTES

Generally speaking, the majority of your carbs should be consumed in two windows: immediately post workout (2–4 hour window) and immediately before bed. This does a number of things, but the most important are that it uses all the carbs for muscle building, not fat storage, and it fuels the overnight muscle building when you are sleeping, which is arguably the most important time in all muscle growth.

The earlier you work out, the harder it is to get the benefits. This makes working out at 6 a.m. really, really tough.

Higher fat pre-workout, lower fat post-workout. Protein should be a constant.

If you must eat breakfast, eat only fat and protein, or, preferably, just protein. Really, though, no one needs breakfast. Your insulin sensitivity is highest in the morning and nearly any carb intake will stop fat burning. Only the skinniest and hardest gainers should ever consider eating before noon, and even they should optimize other aspects before they eat breakfast. Seriously, breakfast just sucks all around.

We can't stress this enough, if you don't work out that day, don't consume carbs. A heavy, strenuous and intense workout does many magical things to your body that allows it to use carbs for muscle building and not fat storage. And this means weights—heavy barbell weights. Running, cardio, sprinting and even working your abs don't cut it.

There is nothing mechanical about this diet. You should very intently listen to your body. Depending on the style, type and intensity of your workout, your carb needs will vary. For instance, a heavy leg workout with squats will probably demand more carbs than an arm workout. This is obvious in hindsight but is helpful to know from the outset. Listen to it day in and day out. Soon you'll start to learn how many carbs you need on any given day.

PROGRAM ADAPTATIONS

The "basic program" is really just a baseline starting point. Everyone is going to be different and have different needs and reactions to the carbs. Some people, like Jason, are much more sensitive to carb intake and need to pay much closer attention to the quantity and type of carbs they ingest. Others, like Brett, can sometimes get away with slightly "trashier" carbs and generally have more fun (think glazed donut sticks).

THIS IS NOT A LOW-CARB DIET

Many people who regularly eat low-carb diets do it not because they are diabetic, but rather they want to take advantage of the very real weight-management benefits of that way of eating. But for our purposes, the very nature of muscle, weight and hormones dictate that you'll need to consume carbs to grow. Embrace carbs—they aren't evil but useful for our goals, and you'll grow to whole new levels!

JASON'S THOUGHTS

Easiest. Diet. Ever. Seriously, there was nothing hard about doing this and I loved every minute of it. Sometimes I might have loved it a bit too much. I experimented with different tweaks and adjustments in the theories I had researched to see what the real-world application would be for me, and over six months I've come down to something I really like. There were times when I wasn't taking the most optimal approach but still getting good gains, and other times when I was gaining too fast. You have to pay attention.

WHAT I DID RIGHT: I didn't get scared by the carbs. I had been a notorious low-carb person for years simply for the easy weight-management aspect of it. Initially I was put off about consuming more carbs, but the more research I did, the more I realized I needed them. There was just no way around it.

WHAT I DID WRONG: There was a point in the middle of the program where I went a bit nuts. I got addicted to the strength gains and I started to drink even more milk, eat more carbs and generally overconsume. I got really, really strong very quickly, but I put on some garbage weight in the form of fat. So I cleaned up my food choices and got my carbs to a more reasonable level and the fat gain stopped. The muscle gains, however, didn't.

My only advice here is that you should use the mirror—it won't lie. If you wake up in the morning tight and solid, your carb levels are probably right on. If you wake up a tad flabby or soft, you overdid it the day before. Cut back on the number and clean up the type of carb a bit and watch the mirror day after day.

To that effect, we offer some program adaptations for people who fall into different categories. So if you want to gain as much weight as possible as quickly as possible or if you are not nearly as carb sensitive, we offer an extreme version. Or, if you want to be sure you are gaining only muscle, are more interested in a slower body recomposition or perhaps are much more sensitive to carbs, we offer a safer variant. Either way the principles are still the same. The variations come with either loosening or tightening of eating windows and types of carbs eaten. In time as you learn the basics and principles, you'll be able to alter the program to suit you individually.

EXTREME PROGRAM VARIATION

Generally speaking, we'll loosen the rules a bit, allowing for more carbs via a longer eating window or suggest you eat the trashiest carbs you can find. Frankly, this is the most fun you can have! This program has the most potential for muscle gains but, if not watched, the most potential fat gain as well. You really shouldn't stay on the extreme program for an indefinite amount of time—we suggest no more than 7 to 10 weeks at a time followed by 1 to 3 weeks of the Basic Program. As we mentioned earlier, it depends on your workouts and your goals, but this is not a year-round nutritional plan. Consider the extreme program a tool for rapid weight (both muscle and fat) gain. Be careful! Know what you are doing and what your goals are!

BRETT'S THOUGHTS

I'll admit I was quite uncomfortable to skip breakfast and then load up on carbs after a workout and keep eating until 8 or 9 p.m. five nights a week. After spending most of the last decade researching and tweaking my diet in order to lose weight, develop a triathlete/marathoner type of body and learn to fuel for events and training, it initially felt like I was throwing everything I'd worked for away. In reality, it wasn't that bad at all. Little did I know that I would enjoy the new routine of eating only after my workouts and reap the benefits from lifting heavier weights than I have ever done before. Let me stress—I've never pushed around this much weight. Ever.

WHAT I DID RIGHT: I followed the program; it's really that easy. I chose which workout and food timing worked for me based on my lifestyle. I have a strange work schedule that changes daily and I try to fit my workouts in while my wife is at work or my daughter at school so I can devote some quality time when they come home. Of course, this is often extremely difficult! The table on page 79 is extremely helpful for me in planning when to eat based on what time I am able to work out.

My biggest victory was defeating that voice in my head that said I couldn't gain muscle or I wouldn't stick with the program and cut out—er, limit—my racing schedule. I was also pretty happy with the way I tweaked my carb intake; for example, when I woke up bloated the following day after a post-workout pepperoni pizza feast, I knew I needed to watch my intake of carbs combined with copious amounts of salt.

WHAT I DID WRONG: During the seven weeks I focused on the routine, there were plenty of times where I didn't pay attention to what and when I was eating and didn't focus on getting the most out of my workouts. My biggest gaffe was not eating enough food post-workout; in order to grow, I needed to consume about an additional 1,000 calories a day and, unless I made a point of keeping a food journal, I would miss my mark. Quite simply, if you don't eat big, you can't grow big.

Every time I slipped up, I got back on track immediately. I've seen first-hand people use the reasoning, "Well, today is already screwed up so I may as well eat whatever I want," and how it inhibits their progress on any routine. It is important to get back on your routine immediately and not wait for tomorrow or next week. There are no cycles for starting and finishing. If you screw up, fix it right away.

Below are suggestions on how to get extreme on top of the normal program. They are in progressive order. Start at the top and work your way down, only adding the next suggestion as you find you need it. Give each suggestion at least a week before you consider adding the next.

1. Make your post-workout eating window at least 4 hours, possibly as high as 6. If you work out after 4 p.m., feel free to go nuts until you go to sleep.

2. All carb sources should be as trashy as possible. We're talking ice cream, donuts, pies, cheesecakes and other fun foods. Did we mention this was going to be fun?

3. Drink a half gallon of whole milk a day. Put milk everywhere!

This should be the stopping point for nearly everyone reading this, and the number of people that would need to go past this step to gain muscle without fat is so slim to be unlikely.

Even so, we'll go further and offer three "extreme-plus" tips:

4. Eat breakfast.

5. Add fat to breakfast.

6. Add carbs to breakfast.

SAFE PROGRAM VARIATION

In direct opposition to the extreme variant, the safe program is going to be about tightening up the eating windows, cleaning up the carb sources and getting more rigorous all around. It isn't nearly as much "fun" as the extreme program but you can safely stay on this program for an indefinite amount of time. The extreme program, as mentioned, is for more short-term gains or to do a rapid bulk.

The safe program is typically the one we use when we go into cruise mode—more for general lifestyle when we want to just live life and make slow, steady gains without worrying about gaining fat. This is a great lifestyle program that also just happens to work well as a body recomposition system.

Below are suggestions on how to get safe on top of the normal program. They are in progressive order. Start at the top and work your way down, only adding the next suggestion as you find you need it. Give each suggestion at least a week before you consider adding the next. Unlike the extreme program, if you wanted to, you could implement all the rules at once.

1. Make your post-workout carb window 2 hours. This means you'll have your post-workout shake and then a high-protein/high-carb meal 1 hour later. You might end the window with another shake. After this, you'll stay pretty clean in your carb sources until bedtime, when you'll have another high-GI carb and protein.

2. All carbs outside of the post-workout shake should be "clean" carbs. This means you'll stick to more complex carbs like sweet potato, brown rice, quinoa or buckwheat.

3. Eliminate all dairy.

4. As a last-ditch effort, eliminate the dextrose in the post-workout shake. This should be the last hi-GI carb in your diet at this point. We consider this an extreme adaptation, one that would significantly slow down your gains.

VEGETARIAN ADAPTATIONS

The true challenge for vegetarians on this muscle-building nutrition plan will be consuming protein. As long as you can find enough protein calories, you'll be fine. If you have no problem with milk, whey protein and/or eggs, this will be quite easy, in fact. Keep away from pasta and bread, which are suboptimal carb sources because of their excess gluten. Stick to rice and potatoes, which are natural—not processed—and somewhat slower-burning sources of carbs.

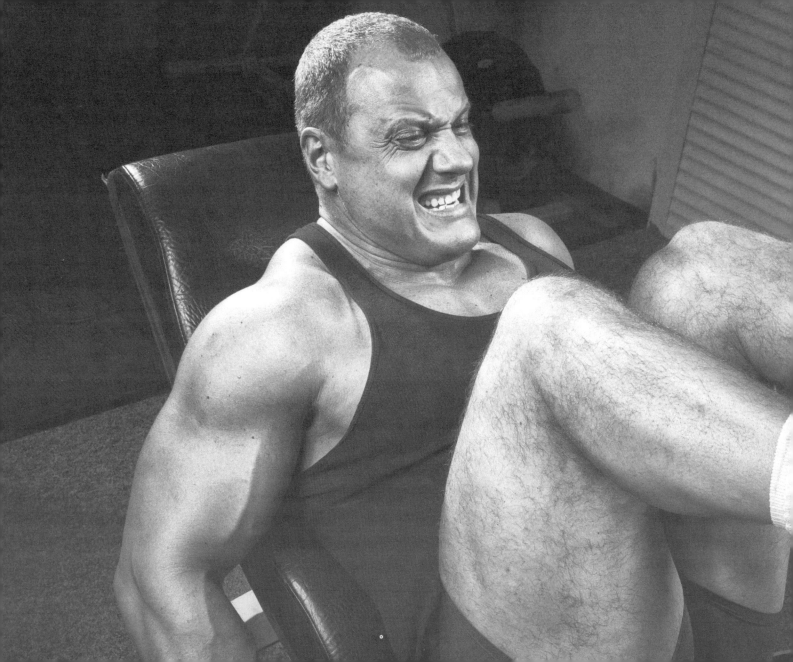

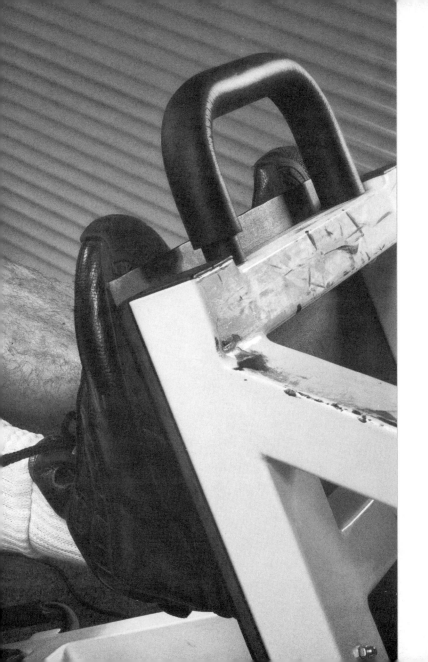

PART IV:
THE KITCHEN

What to Eat

The following are our top-10 picks for the leanest and healthiest protein sources, in order of highest to lowest lean-protein content (per cup, where possible, and per serving in ounces elsewhere) *and* best overall nutritional value. (Each selection has a corresponding recipe in "Cook Your Way to Big Muscles" on page 92).

1. NUT BUTTERS: Nut butters such as peanut or almond butter are excellent sources of protein, containing 65 g protein per cup and 56 g protein per cup, respectively. (Compare this to their whole form: peanuts contain 36 g protein per cup; raw almonds contain 32 g protein per cup.) Nut butters do contain a decent amount of fat, but it's heart-healthy fat. Also, the typical serving of nut butter is 2 tablespoons and not 1 cup, so if you eat nut butters in moderation (and also save them for non-workout days when you'll be eating more fat), they are still a great choice. Corresponding recipe: Cold Sesame Noodles (page 95).

2. LEAN TURKEY BREAST: While whole, roasted turkey breast contains around 52 g protein per cup, it also contains a lot of fat! A great alternative is lean ground turkey breast as it cuts down considerably on the fat content, while still containing 34.5 g protein per cup. With the leanest products containing only 0.5–1.5 g fat per cup, lean ground turkey breast is one of the leanest selections on this list. Corresponding recipe: Cheat Sheet Chili (page 98).

3. CHICKEN BREAST (SKINLESS): Chicken breast has about 46 g per cup (or 30 g protein per 3.5 oz.). Poultry also has the highest amount of valine, one of the three branched-chain amino acids (BCAA) essential to muscle building, at 2,500–5,000 mg of valine per 1 pound of meat! Corresponding recipe: Tequila-Lime Chicken Fajitas (page 97).

4. TUNA: Tuna is one of the leanest, highest-protein seafood selections you can make. Its protein content ranges according to the cut, preparation and other factors. Of all the kinds of tuna, bluefin and yellowfin tuna typically have the highest protein contents. Generic canned tuna (packed in water) typically contains about 35–39 g protein per cup. Corresponding recipe: Samurai Salad (Wasabi Tuna Steak Salad) (page 94).

5. LEAN DAIRY SELECTIONS: Some of the best high-protein dairy choices include hard cheeses, particularly Parmesan and Asiago, which are not only high in protein but also low in fat. Of all of the hard cheeses, shredded Parmesan cheese is the highest in protein at 38.5 g protein per cup, closely followed by Pecorino Romano and Asiago, both at 32 g protein per cup.

Cottage cheese is another great option: out of all the different kinds of cottage cheese, 1% milk fat cottage cheese is the highest in protein at 28 g per cup. Next highest is 2% milk fat cottage cheese at 27 g protein per cup (4% milk fat, small-curd cottage cheese is 25 g protein per cup). Cottage cheese is 80% casein protein and 20% whey protein, which is a highly effective combination. Here's why: to build muscle in the most rapid, efficient manner, you need to slow the rate of protein breakdown in the body while accelerating protein synthesis. Casein accomplishes the former function and whey the latter.

Corresponding recipe: No-Brainer Eggplant & Zucchini Lasagna (page 96). It contains three super high-protein cheeses: cottage cheese, Parmesan and mozzarella (part-skim mozzarella is 29 g protein per cup; whole-milk mozzarella is 25.1 g protein per cup). The recipe also calls for eggs (24 g protein per cup, cooked) to help you nourish and grow your muscle mass as you follow this book's exercise program. All that protein will really help you to pack on the muscle!

6. WHOLE SEEDS & NUTS: Some of the highest-protein selections in this category include shelled pumpkin seeds (36 g protein per cup), flaxseeds (31 g protein per cup) and sesame seeds (25.4 g protein per cup), all of which can be found in the corresponding recipe: Almond-Cherry-Sesame Crunch Bars (page 93).

7. WHEY PROTEIN ISOLATE: Whey protein isolate (WPI) is 25 g per 1 ounce if you go with a product that contains a 90% protein-concentration level. Please note that protein content and concentration can vary by brand. Corresponding recipe: Protein Recovery Shake (page 95). This recipe also contains whole milk, which has 8 g protein per cup.

8. TOFU: Tofu's protein content can be 22–26 g per cup, depending upon the variety you purchase (soft, firm, extra-firm, etc.). Typically, the firmer the tofu, the higher in protein. Corresponding recipe: Creamy Red Hot Pepper Dip (page 93).

9. WILD SALMON: Salmon is packed with omega-3s and protein, at 23 g protein per cup. Tip: For the highest protein and omega-3 content, buy wild salmon instead of farm-raised. In comparison to farm-raised salmon, wild salmon contains more omega-3s and is 20% higher in protein but 20% lower in fat. Corresponding recipe: Teriyaki Salmon Burgers (page 97).

10. LEAN BEEF: Protein content varies with cut. London broil is one of the leanest cuts of beef, containing around 25 g protein and 9 g fat per 4-ounce serving. Top round of beef (or veal) provides a decent amount of protein at around 31 g per 3-ounce serving. Lean ground beef contains around 23 g protein per 4-ounce serving. Corresponding recipes: Steak Kebabs (page 94) and Shepherd's Pie (page 98).

Sample 3-Day Muscle-Building Meal Plan

To help you pack on the muscle, below is three days' worth of simple, easy-to-prepare meals and snacks. No, it's not the same thing every day. There's lots of variety, and the food choices can be switched around to produce many different meal combinations.

This plan is going to use the 12–3 p.m. workout schedule as a template/example, but feel free to tailor meals to suit whichever eating protocol schedule you'll be using.

Remember: For pre-workout meals, eat protein and fat, but limit carbs. For post-workout meals and snacks, eat lots of protein and carbs, but limit fat. Protein consumption is always a constant.

Mix and match some of these food ideas and do a little homework. Fire up your trusty Internet browser and track down some other recipes that meet the simple pre- and post-workout nutrient criteria on page 79 in "7-Week Muscle-Build Nutrition Plan."

No time to make your own meals? Open up a can or pouch (even two) of tuna and flake it over some chopped romaine lettuce and veggies. Or throw a turkey burger on the grill and just forgo the bun pre-workout; you can even top it with an egg lightly fried in a teaspoon of coconut oil. With even a little bit of creativity, you can create meals that fuel your muscles, give you the energy you need to work out, and still be able to eat normal foods without suffering. As far as dietary modifications go, the ones in this book are relatively easy to adapt to your daily life.

3-Day Muscle-Building Meal Plan

	MONDAY (Workout Day)	TUESDAY (Non-Workout Day)	WEDNESDAY (Workout Day)
Meal 1	light pre-workout meal: Samurai Salad (Wasabi Tuna Steak Salad) (page 94)	Steak Kebabs (page 94)	light pre-workout meal: Creamy Red Hot Pepper Dip (page 93) served with raw vegetable slices
Post-Workout Shake	Protein Recovery Shake (page 95)	--	Blend together 2 c. chocolate milk, 1 scoop whey protein isolate and 2 Tbsp. malt
Meal 2	Cheat Sheet Chili (page 98) served with baked tortilla chips	Broiled scallops in a butter–white wine sauce with a side of yellow squash, zucchini and red bell peppers	Tequila-Lime Chicken Fajitas (page 97)
Meal 3/Snack	Teriyaki Salmon Burgers (page 97) served with a baked sweet potato OR fruit and yogurt with honey	Chicken breast and steamed spinach tossed in extra-virgin olive oil, lemon juice, salt and pepper, and a dash of crushed red chili pepper flakes OR Almond-Cherry-Sesame Crunch Bars (page 93)	Cold Sesame Noodles (page 95)
Meal 4/Snack	Shepherd's Pie (page 98) OR vanilla or chocolate pudding	--	No-Brainer Eggplant & Zucchini Lasagna (page 96)

Cook Your Way to Big Muscles

Each of the following recipes corresponds to the earlier list of the top-10 lean-protein sources in the "What to Eat" chapter (page 86). These recipes have been grouped by pre- and post-workout foods to indicate when you should eat them to maximize muscle gain. Now that you know how the recipes fit into the nutrition program, let's bring on the food!

Pre-Workout Recipes

Creamy Red Hot Pepper Dip

This dip recipe is perfect for parties and casual get-togethers, or just eat it as a snack. Not only is this recipe high in protein (1 c. firm tofu has 22–26 g. protein!), but the capsaicin in the red chili pepper flakes has a plethora of health benefits: it fights inflammation, provides natural pain relief, boosts immunity, speeds up metabolism and aids in respiratory, cardiovascular and digestive health. And, on top of all that, it takes practically zero time to prepare.   YIELD: 1 CUP

½ c. roasted red bell pepper strips, drained (from a jar)
6 oz. firm tofu
3 Tbsp. freshly squeezed lemon juice
½ tsp. garlic powder
½ tsp. onion powder
¼ tsp. dried parsley
¼ tsp. dried oregano

¼ tsp. dried basil
¼ tsp. dried marjoram
¼ tsp. dried thyme
¼ tsp. salt, or to taste
⅛ tsp. red chili pepper flakes (for mild heat), or to taste

Combine all ingredients in a food processor and pulse until smooth. Transfer to a small serving dish, cover and refrigerate for at least 30 minutes to allow flavors to meld and dip to thicken just a bit. Serve with raw, sliced vegetables or other low-carb accompaniment.

TIP: Why should you have dried apricots, dates, bananas and pineapple on hand? Because they're packed with vitamin A and potassium, both of which can really boost your testosterone levels. See "Maxing Your T" on page 26.

Almond-Cherry-Sesame Crunch Bars

Build big muscles with these healthy, high-protein snack bars! They've got almonds, pumpkin seeds, almond butter, sesame seeds and flaxseed. Of course, flaxseeds are also a great source of Omega-3s, which help reduce post-exercise inflammation. Per ¼ c. serving, pumpkin seeds, flaxseeds and almonds each have 8 g of protein, while sesame seeds have 6.36 g. Almond butter has 7 g of protein per 2 Tbsp. serving. These nuts and seeds contain heart-healthy monounsaturated fats, which, in combination with their protein and carbohydrate content, will really satisfy your hunger and fill you up. A little goes a long way, so easy does it. You'll be surprised how filling one bar really is.   YIELD: ABOUT 12 BARS (1 BAR = 1 SERVING)

⅔ c. sliced almonds
⅔ c. shelled pumpkin seeds
½ c. ground flaxseed
½ c. brown or white sesame seeds
1 c. no-sugar-added dried cherries (Whole Foods Market carries these)
2 tsp. pure vanilla extract

½ c. pure maple syrup
¼ c. extra-virgin coconut oil
¼ c. almond butter
2 tsp. ground cinnamon
½ tsp. ground allspice
½ tsp. salt

Preheat oven to 350°F. Line an 11 x 7-in. metal baking pan with parchment paper. Combine all ingredients in a medium bowl and fold together until thoroughly mixed. Pour into the prepared pan and spread mixture until the pan is completely covered, pressing down gently to compact the mixture a bit (to about ½-in. thickness). Bake for about 35 minutes, or until golden brown. Allow to cool completely, about 10–15 minutes. Then, while the bars are still in the pan, cut into 12 bars. Chill in the refrigerator for at least 1–2 hours to allow bars to set; this will help the bars firm up. Transfer the bars to a serving plate using a small spatula (they should easily lift from the pan). Store the remainder in an airtight container for future snacking. Serve and enjoy!

Steak Kebabs

YIELD: 6–8 KEBABS ON 12-INCH SKEWERS

Marinade:
1 c. extra-virgin olive oil
5 Tbsp. freshly squeezed lemon juice
1 Tbsp. paprika
2 tsp. ground cumin
1 tsp. onion powder
1 tsp. garlic powder
1 tsp. ground coriander
½ tsp. ground allspice
½ tsp. ground black pepper
1 tsp. salt

Kebab:
8 oz. top sirloin steak, trimmed of fat and
   silver skin removed, and cut into
   1½-in.cubes
1 c. red onion (½ medium onion)
1 c. green bell pepper (1 small pepper)
1 c. red bell pepper (1 small pepper)
1 (8-oz.) whole box mushrooms
½ pint whole cherry tomatoes,
1½ c. pineapple chunks, cut into 1½-in.
   cubes

Pour all marinade ingredients into a small bowl and mix until thoroughly combined. Next, place the steak cubes into a medium bowl and the vegetables and fruit in a separate, large bowl. Pour a ½ c. of the marinade over the steak and the remaining amount over the vegetables and fruit. Toss each separate bowl with separate utensils. Refrigerate until serving time. (The marinating can be done up to a day in advance; it's easiest to do the prep the night before and just let the kebab ingredients marinate overnight.) About 30 minutes before serving time, spear all of the kebab ingredients onto 12-in. skewers, alternating the steak cubes with the fruits and vegetables. Be sure to leave enough room at the tips of the skewers so that you can easily grasp them. Grill on medium-high heat, until the steak reaches the desired level of doneness, anywhere from 5–15 minutes. (Test a piece of steak with a knife and fork.) Kebabs should have grill marks on them when ready.

Samurai Salad (Wasabi Tuna Steak Salad)

YIELD: 4 SERVINGS

Marinade:
6 Tbsp. (⅜ c.) sesame oil
2 Tbsp. freshly squeezed lime juice
2 Tbsp. soy sauce
½ tsp. wasabi paste
2 tsp. ground ginger
2 tsp. garlic powder
¼ tsp. kosher salt
½ tsp. coarsely ground black pepper
2 Tbsp. sesame seeds

Salad:
1 lb. very fresh tuna steak, cut into 1-in.-
   thick cubes
1 ripe medium Haas avocado, peeled,
   pitted and sliced into bite-size pieces
¼ c. scallions, sliced crosswise into
   ⅛-in.-thick rounds (about 4
   scallions)
½ c. diced red onion
¼ c. roughly chopped cilantro leaves

1 heart of romaine lettuce, chopped into
   bite-sized pieces
¾ c. diced red bell pepper
¼ c. shredded carrots
¾ c. sliced cucumbers, peel scored
   vertically with the tines of a fork and
   then sliced crosswise into ¼-in.-
   thick rounds

Salad Dressing:
¼ c. sesame oil
2 Tbsp. soy sauce
2 Tbsp. freshly squeezed lime juice
1 Tbsp. water
1 Tbsp. honey
1 tsp. ground ginger
1 tsp. garlic powder
¼ tsp. ground mustard
½ Tbsp. sesame seeds
⅛ tsp. ground black pepper

Combine all marinade ingredients in a small bowl and whisk until emulsified. Place tuna cubes in a resealable plastic bag along with marinade, and seal bag. Massage marinade into the tuna from outside of the bag until well-coated. Let rest on countertop until tuna reaches room temperature, 20–30 minutes. In the meantime, place the remaining salad ingredients in a large salad bowl and toss. Next, combine all the salad dressing ingredients in a small bowl, whisk until emulsified and set aside. Place a large wok or stir-fry pan over high heat; make sure the pan is very hot before adding tuna cubes. Cook tuna cubes on high heat for only 30 seconds per side (i.e., cook on all six sides). (Cover wok with a splatter screen to avoid getting zinged with bursts of crackling, sizzling hot oil.) Set cooked tuna aside on a plate to cool, then transfer them to the salad bowl. Drizzle salad with salad dressing and gently toss. Serve and enjoy!

Chef's Notes: Both the marinade and the salad dressing can be made in advance to save time. To avoid cross-contamination, be sure to wash your hands after handling raw fish.

Post-Workout Recipes

Protein Recovery Shake

This shake contains the ideal mix of muscle-building elements:
1. Easily digestible contents (in liquid or pulverized form).
By making this shake in a blender, you're breaking down solids into liquids, which means your body doesn't have to do that work and thus more quickly absorbs the nutrients. ***2. Lean, high-protein sources containing all-three branched-chain amino acids (leucine, isoleucine and valine) and omega-3 fatty acids.***
The first aids in protein synthesis while the latter helps reduce post-exercise inflammation. ***3. Fast-acting, high-GI/GL carbs.***
These carbs favor pure glucose sources to aid in the production of insulin in order to quickly move nutrients to muscles and vital organs. ***4. Minimal fat.*** *Minimal post-exercise fat intake is generally recommended, unless you're having trouble gaining weight.* ***5. Alkalizing (i.e., acid-buffering) ingredients.***
These aid in muscle tissue repair and recovery, and thus counter the effects of a high-intensity workout. Alkalizing foods help build muscle, whereas acidizing foods actually break it down.

6. Antioxidants. *Antioxidants remove toxic free-radicals that interfere with muscle-building (and can actually cause muscle damage).* YIELD: ABOUT 24 OZ. OR 3 (1-C.) SERVINGS

½ c. crushed ice

¼ c. deglet noor dates (i.e., common dates)

¼ c. dried Turkish apricots (i.e., common apricots)

1 large banana, quartered

1 pint (2 c.) red raspberries

⅓ c. whey protein isolate powder (about 1 scoop)

1 pint (2 c.) milk

¼ c. pineapple juice (not from concentrate)

1 Tbsp. honey

Add all solid ingredients to a blender first, followed by liquid ingredients and pulse until smooth and creamy. Pour into glasses and drink up!

Cold Sesame Noodles

YIELD: 2 SERVINGS

Main Course:

6–8 c. water

4 oz. soba (buckwheat) noodles (2 servings)

½ c. julienned carrots

½ c. julienned seedless cucumber (about ½ large cucumber)

2 Tbsp. scallions

2 Tbsp. roughly chopped fresh cilantro, densely packed

Peanut Sauce:

½ c. creamy-style peanut butter

½ Tbsp. minced garlic (about 4 medium cloves)

1-in. piece fresh ginger (peel using the side of a spoon), minced (about ½ Tbsp.)

½ tsp. salt, or to taste

pinch of red chili pepper flakes

1 Tbsp. finely minced fresh cilantro, densely packed

½ Tbsp. freshly squeezed lime juice

1 Tbsp. soy sauce

2 Tbsp. honey

1 Tbsp. sesame seed oil

¼ c. light unsweetened coconut milk (from a can)

2 Tbsp. water, or more, if needed

½ Tbsp. sesame seeds

In a medium stockpot over high heat, bring water to a boil, add soba noodles and cook for about 4 minutes, until al dente. Pour noodles into colander over sink, rinse with cold water and drain. Transfer to a large bowl and set aside. Wash out pot. Combine all peanut sauce ingredients in a food processor and pulse until smooth. (This step can be done in advance.) In the same pot you used for the noodles, cook peanut sauce for 3–4 minutes over medium-low heat, or until raw garlic smell disappears, stirring continuously. (Add more water as needed to prevent burning the bottom of the sauce and achieve desired consistency.) Gently fold in sesame seeds and then pour sauce into the bowl with noodles. Add carrots, cucumbers, scallions and cilantro, and toss until all noodles have been evenly coated with sauce.

No-Brainer Eggplant & Zucchini Lasagna

This super-easy recipe might be easy to make, but it'll taste like you've been slaving over a hot oven for hours. A few minor shortcuts—like using jarred tomato sauce and oven-ready lasagna noodles—will prepare a quick and nutritious meal. YIELD: ABOUT 12 SERVINGS

Lasagna Filling:
4 c. cottage cheese (32 oz. container)
2 large eggs, beaten
½ tsp. salt
½ tsp. ground black pepper
⅛ tsp. ground nutmeg
½ c. grated fresh Parmigiano-Reggiano cheese

Lasagna Assembly:
extra-virgin olive oil, for spraying or brushing the baking dish

1 (8 oz.) box 12 no-bake lasagna noodles
2 (24 oz.) jars no-sugar-added tomato sauce
2 medium zucchini, sliced lengthwise into ⅛-in.-thick strips (about 14 oz. total)
1 large eggplant, sliced lengthwise into ⅛-in.-thick thick strips (about 16 oz. total)
1 (8 oz.) bag shaved or grated fresh Parmigiano-Reggiano cheese
1 c. shredded mozzarella cheese

With a spray bottle or pastry brush, lightly coat a 9 x 13-in. glass baking dish with extra-virgin olive oil and set aside. Place on top of an 11 x 17-in. rimmed glass baking dish covered with aluminum foil to prevent drips and keep your oven clean— lasagna tends to get rather bubbly when it bakes. In a food processor, purée all filling ingredients together until well-blended and smooth. Transfer to a bowl. Cover and refrigerate for at least 1 hour to allow flavors to meld. (You can do this step in advance if you prefer.)

Preheat oven to 375°F. Remove bowl containing the cheese filling from the refrigerator. Assemble lasagna in the glass baking dish: ladle about 1 cup of the filling into the dish and, using a spatula, evenly spread a thin layer of it the across the bottom so that it's completely covered with filling. Next, add a layer of 3 evenly spaced lasagna noodles vertically across the longer side of the dish, followed by a layer of tomato sauce and then a layer of alternating zucchini and eggplant strips. Be sure to fill in any gaps with any smaller pieces of zucchini or eggplant; to fill in the holes, cut them into smaller pieces if needed. Also, make sure you leave enough filling for the final layer, or else you'll be scraping the heck out of the bowl to eke out the last little bits. Repeat until you've reached the final layer of sauce. Then sprinkle a layer of mozzarella on top, completely covering the surface of the dish with cheese. Cover baking dish with aluminum foil and bake for 30 minutes. Then remove the foil and continue baking, uncovered, until the top is golden brown and the filling is bubbling, about 15 more minutes. Remove from the oven and let rest 10–15 minutes before cutting. Sprinkle Parmigiano-Reggiano cheese evenly over the top, cut into 12 squares and serve.

Chef's Note: Since tomato reacts unfavorably with metal, it's best to use a glass baking dish rather than a metal one (including disposable aluminum pans).

Tequila-Lime Chicken Fajitas

YIELD: 4–6 SERVINGS

Marinade:

1 lb. thinly sliced, boneless, skinless, chicken breasts, washed and trimmed of fat

1 tsp. garlic powder

½ Tbsp. mild Mexican chili powder

2 Tbsp. paprika

½ Tbsp. dried oregano

¼ tsp. salt

1 tsp. grated lime zest (from 1 large lime)

3 Tbsp. freshly squeezed lime juice (from 1 large lime)

¼ c. gold tequila

Other Fajita Ingredients:

1 Tbsp. extra-virgin olive oil

1 c. sliced yellow onion, halved and then cut into ½-in.-thick crescent slivers (about ½ medium onion)

1 c. sliced red bell pepper, seeded and sliced into long, ½-in.-thick strips (about ½ large pepper)

1 c. green bell pepper, seeded and sliced into long, ½-in.-thick strips (about ½ large pepper)

¼ c. gold tequila

4–6 medium soft flour tortillas

Toppings:

pico de gallo (or salsa)

4–6 Tbsp. shredded Monterey Jack cheese

4–6 Tbsp. Greek yogurt, about 1 Tbsp. per fajita

a few avocado slices or guacamole

2 Tbsp. finely minced fresh cilantro, for garnish

Place chicken on an even, non-porous surface, cut on the bias into 1 x 3-in. strips, and transfer to a resealable plastic bag. Next, add remaining marinade ingredients to the bag, seal and refrigerate overnight or for at least 6–8 hours. Sauté onions in extra-virgin olive oil over medium heat in a large sauté pan until translucent, about 3 minutes. Then add green and red bell peppers and cook for about 3 more minutes, or until onions turn golden brown and the peppers become tender. Deglaze with remaining ¼ c. tequila and cook for another 3–4 minutes, until liquid reduces to a thin layer on the bottom of the pan. Remove from heat, transfer to a medium bowl, and set aside. Heat the same pan over high heat. Sauté chicken in the residual olive oil and marinade juices for about 3 minutes per side, or until tender and the meat is no longer pink on the inside. (Chicken will cook very quickly as the pan should be very hot at this point, so make sure you watch the chicken very carefully!) Transfer to a clean bowl and set aside. Next, assemble fajitas: Divide the chicken into equal portions. Place a small amount of chicken on each tortilla, then add onions, peppers and any other toppings you'd like. Serve and enjoy!

Teriyaki Salmon Burgers

YIELD: 2 BURGERS

Salmon Patty:

1 (7.5 oz.) can wild Alaskan salmon packed in water, drained and flaked

½ c. unflavored bread crumbs

1 large egg

½ tsp. onion powder

½ tsp. garlic powder

1 tsp. sesame oil

¼ tsp. ground mustard

1 tsp. ground ginger

1 Tbsp. white or brown sesame seeds

1 Tbsp. freshly squeezed lemon juice

2 tsp. teriyaki sauce (or if unavailable, soy sauce will work)

⅛ tsp. ground black pepper (or, for more heat, substitute ⅛ tsp. red chili pepper flakes)

Burger Assembly:

2 whole wheat burger buns

lettuce

2 large tomato slices

2 red onion ring slices (raw or grilled)

tartar sauce (or other preferred sauce)

Place all salmon patty ingredients in a medium bowl, mash salmon, and then mix together until thoroughly combined. Make into two ½-in.-thick patties, place on a plate, and refrigerate in a covered container for at least 30 minutes to let flavors meld. Open the grill and lightly spray the grill grate with olive oil to prevent patties from sticking. Then set the grill to medium-high heat. Place patties onto the hot grill and cook for 3–5 minutes per side, or until desired level of doneness has been reached. Remove from the grill and place on buns. Add desired toppings and sauce, and serve.

Cheat Sheet Chili

This flavorful, low-fat turkey chili recipe—made without adding any additional oil!—will help turn you into a lean, mean, muscle-building machine! YIELD: 4–6 SERVINGS

1 lb. lean ground turkey (or, to go even leaner, use lean ground turkey breast)

2 c. water, divided

1 (8 oz.) can unflavored, crushed tomatoes

1 (6 oz.) can tomato paste

1 (15.5 oz.) can black beans, drained and rinsed

1 (15.5 oz.) can kidney beans, drained and rinsed

1 c. green bell pepper, coarsely chopped

1 c. red bell pepper, coarsely chopped

1 Tbsp. apple cider vinegar

1 large bay leaf

2 Tbsp. paprika

1 Tbsp. ground cumin

2 tsp. onion powder

2 tsp. garlic salt

1 tsp. ground oregano

1 tsp. ground coriander

1 tsp. ground cinnamon, or to taste

⅛ tsp. cayenne pepper, or to taste

2 Tbsp. masa (corn) flour

¼ c. roughly chopped fresh cilantro leaves, roughly chopped, for garnish (about 1 Tbsp. per person)

In a large stockpot, sear ground turkey over high heat for 10–12 minutes or until browned, stirring continually to break up meat and evenly brown it. Remove from heat and drain any excess liquid fat using a pan drainer. Return to high heat. Add 1 c. water, followed by crushed tomatoes, tomato paste, black beans, kidney beans, green and red bell peppers, apple cider vinegar, and all dried spices. Stir together to combine, then reduce heat to low. Cover with a tightly fitting lid and simmer for 20 minutes, or until meat is tender. Lift lid to check on chili every couple of minutes, stirring occasionally and adding more water when

necessary. After 20 minutes, remove lid and stir in masa and remaining 1 c. water. Cook for an additional 10–15 minutes, or until desired thickness has been reached. (When chili is finished cooking, bell peppers should still retain their color and a bit of their crunch.) Remove from heat and let cool for 10–15 minutes before serving. Discard bay leaf. Garnish with fresh cilantro and serve.

Shepherd's Pie

The perfect mix of high-protein, high-carb, low-fat elements for a hearty post-workout meal. YIELD: 4–6 SERVINGS

Mashed Potato Topping:

3 qts. (12 c.) lightly salted water (for boiling potatoes)

4 large red-skinned potatoes, peeled (makes about 2 c. mashed)

2 Tbsp. unsalted butter, at room temperature

¼ tsp. salt, or to taste

¼ tsp. ground black pepper, or to taste

2 Tbsp. whole milk

½ c. skim milk

1 egg

¼ c. grated Parmigiano-Reggiano cheese

Filling:

1 lb. lean ground (or minced) beef or lamb

1 Tbsp. extra-virgin olive oil

1 c. shredded yellow onion (1 small onion)

¼ c. shredded shallots

1 Tbsp. finely minced garlic (about 2 large cloves)

½ c. red wine

¼ c. Worcestershire sauce

¼ c. tomato paste

¼ tsp. salt, or to taste

¼ tsp. ground black pepper, or to taste

¼ tsp. ground nutmeg

2 tsp. paprika

1 ½ c. low-sodium reduced-fat chicken or beef broth, divided

½ c. shredded carrots

2 Tbsp. fresh Italian flat-leaf parsley, densely packed and finely minced

1 Tbsp. fresh rosemary, densely packed and finely minced

1 Tbsp. fresh thyme, densely packed

IMPORTANT: Drinking milk is a great method for gaining weight in general, as it provides a massive amount of nutrients to help you rapidly grow muscle. So which kind of milk should you drink after your workout? Well, that depends upon your exact goals and current progress with respect to weight gain and muscle mass. Having trouble gaining? Keep pounding the whole milk. Gaining muscle just fine? Drink skim or 1 percent if you want to be extra careful about not gaining fat. Gaining a bit too much? Scale it back to skim milk. Please note that this is a strategy for post-workout consumption. You'll still need to consume some fat, especially on your days off. Post-workout food should generally be high-carb, high-protein and low-fat, but the fat content should correspond to your individual needs.

Bring the lightly salted water to a rolling boil in a large sauce/stock pot, about 8 minutes. Meanwhile, in a large (12–13-in.) sauté pan, sear beef or lamb on high heat (without oil) until browned, 5–7 minutes, stirring frequently. Stir to break up meat into small, bite-size bits. Remove from heat and discard any residual fat. Using a slotted spoon, transfer into a metal colander to allow the excess liquid and any remaining fat to drain. Set aside. By now, water should be at a rolling boil. Add potatoes to the pot, then set your kitchen timer for 20–25 minutes.

Make the filling: In the same sauté pan you used to sear the meat, heat olive oil on low heat until it glistens. Then add onion, shallots and garlic and cook until tender, about 5 minutes. Just as ingredients start to brown, deglaze pan with red wine and Worcestershire sauce. Stir continuously with a spatula to break up any of the fond (i.e., the brown bits) that have stuck to the bottom and sides of the pan. Immediately return drained meat to the pan and stir in tomato paste until thoroughly combined. (Do this step quickly before all of the liquid disappears.) Quickly season with salt and pepper, ground nutmeg and paprika, and then add ¾ c. of the chicken or beef broth to the pan, stirring continuously. Turn up heat to high and cook for about 10 minutes, or until liquid is almost completely absorbed. Stir in carrots and another ½ c. broth, and continue to cook for another 5 minutes. Add remaining ¼ c. broth and parsley, rosemary and thyme, and cook until liquid has been reduced to a thin layer on the bottom of the pan, 3–5 more minutes. Remove from heat and allow to cool.

Make the mashed potato topping: Drain water from pot of potatoes and let them cool for 5–10 minutes. In the same pot, mash potatoes until creamy and smooth, or pass through a potato ricer or Mouli grater. Place butter in the bottom of the pot containing the potatoes, turn on the heat to high, and cook for 30–60 seconds, or until butter starts to melt. Quickly remove from heat, season with salt and pepper, stir in whole and skim milk, and whisk in egg. Mix until just combined and set aside. (Be careful not to overmix mashed potatoes or else they'll become glue-like and unappetizing in terms of both taste and texture.)

Assemble pie: Preheat oven to 400°F. Put the meat filling into a 1½-qt. circular ovenproof glass baking bowl (or deep pie plate), and then top with the mashed potato topping, using the back of a large spoon. The mashed potato mixture should form a slight mound on top of the bowl, as the pie will deflate slightly after baking. Sprinkle with Parmigiano-Reggiano cheese, making sure to evenly spread the cheese so that it covers the entire surface of the mashed potatoes. Use a fork to prick the top so that the potato mixture forms little peaks on its surface. Bake for 30–40 minutes, or until bubbling and golden brown. Divide into equal portions, transfer to plates and serve immediately.

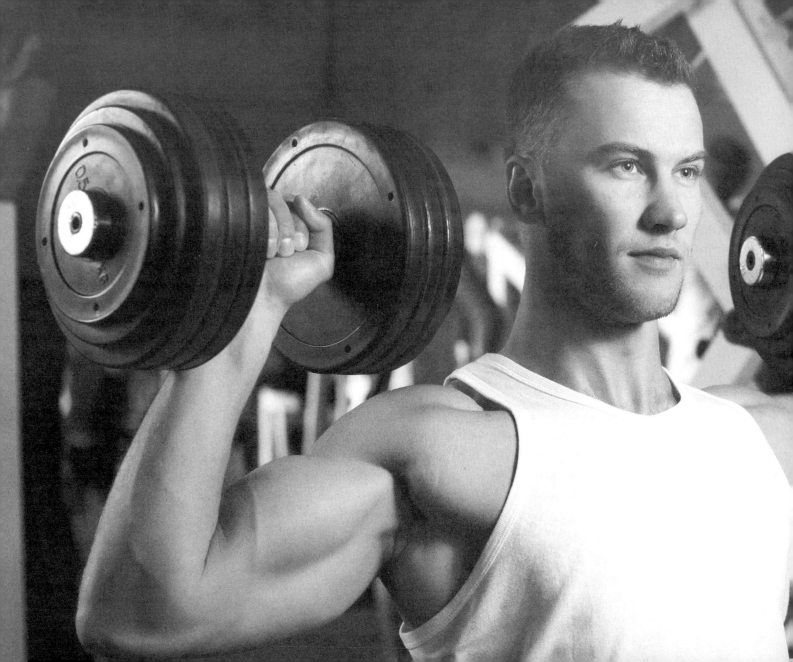

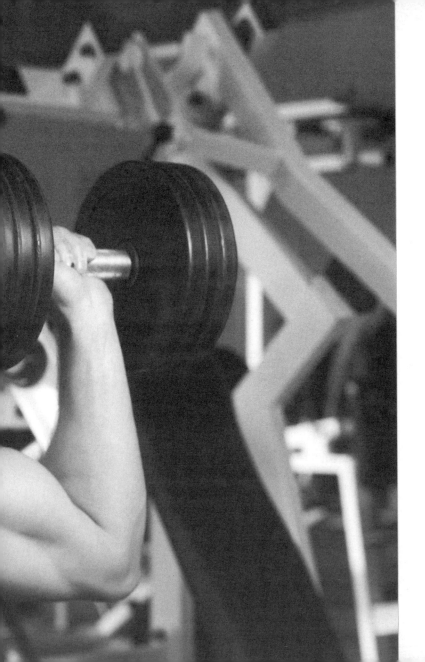

PART V: EXERCISES

Lifting Basics

All the lifts, exercises and movements in this book should be done in the strictest fashion. No bouncing weights, no sloppy form—you'll only be cheating yourself and potentially tearing muscles or tendons.

Your goal is gaining muscle size and mass, and to achieve that goal we want as much muscle activation as possible, not the greatest weight lifted possible (these are different goals). Keep this in mind at all times. You may need to check your ego at the door; you will be performing workouts with considerably less than your 1RM (one rep max) weight on the bar. Remember that you're not going to the gym to impress anyone with your lifts, you're doing it to grow muscle—you can impress more folks with those later.

Don't Screw Up Your Workout

The quickest way to sabotage your workout is to lift too heavy, too fast. The resulting soreness will knock you off track faster than you can say DOMS (delayed onset muscle soreness). Take it easy on your first few workouts: use light weights—or none at all—and focus on perfecting your form before you add weight. Check your ego. It's not about lifting the most you can; it's about doing it properly. You can't grow muscles when you're stuck in bed with extremely sore quads and glutes or a pulled muscle, right?

Post-Workout Routine

After a workout, your first plan of attack to build those muscles is to eat and flood your muscles with the nutritional building blocks they need to repair and grow. But you also need to relax and recover in order for that to take place. Post-workout, take it as easy as you can. This means you're not jumping on a treadmill or playing some pick-up hoops. To hit your growth goals, you need to give your body adequate down-time to build.

In order to combat soreness, some athletes will take an ice bath immediately after a workout. They swear by the reduced soreness the next day; others say it's nonsense. Decide for yourself by taking a long, cold shower after an upper-body workout, or soak in a cold tub (add ice only if you can handle it!) after squat and Deadlift days. Some reports show as much as a 50 percent reduction in DOMS the day following a hard workout, and if it keeps you on track, it's completely worth the chill!

The Big Four

There are four basic compound movements that should be the core of your workout. These movements—barbell squat, barbell deadlift, barbell overhead press and barbell bench press—together work the entire body and stress it into growth. These movements involve multiple muscles across multiple joints, hence the name "compound." Each has many variations and substitutions, but there's nothing like the original!

BARBELL SQUATS

The granddaddy of all exercises, the barbell squat. Do a quick Internet search for old-school lifting, and I'm sure the squat is at the top of the search results. The squat has been around forever and been both revered and vilified in that time. The squat also elicits more fear and angst than any other exercise on the planet. Chances are if someone is going to skip a day at the gym, that day "just happens" to include squats.

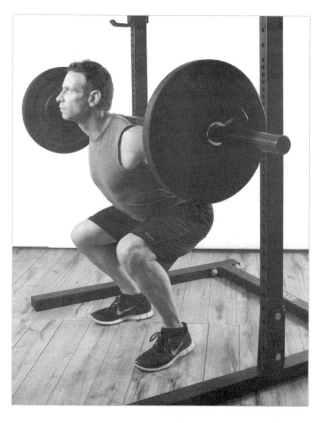

Why the hate? Why the avoidance? Simple! Squats. Are. Hard. They work nearly your entire body, take balance and coordination, and can have you crying in just a few reps even with lighter weights. Add some real weight to the bar and work through a full squat set and you'll feel like you just sprinted a mile. Squats are key to pack muscle all over your body but require perfect form in order to prevent injury and reap the benefits.

But they work. And they work like no other exercise (except the deadlift, more on that later). Your lower body makes up more than half of your total large muscle mass. Squats blast your entire lower body in one powerful movement. You'll be working your quads, hamstrings, glutes and hip flexors all in one go. Additionally, your core will get blasted as you control the bar on the way down and up, and your upper back will be used to stabilize the bar on your traps. One movement, nearly your entire body involved.

Squats should be your number-one lift. Never, ever skip a day you are doing squats. If you want to put on muscle—anywhere on your body—make sure to keep squats in your workout. Bigger arms, shoulders and upper back? The squat is key. Why? Multi-joint, multi-muscle movements like squats and deadlifts (the two biggies) not only work myriad muscles all over your body, they also release more of the juice that helps you build muscles, get pumped and stay lean: testosterone. See "Maxing Your T" on page 26.

Absolutely, positively start with bodyweight squats to master the proper technique before you even touch a weight. Progress through a broomstick, a length of PVC pipe and eventually an Olympic bar without any weight before you start to slide any plates on. Did we make that clear enough?

BARBELL DEADLIFTS

There's a reason that squats and deadlifts make up two of the three traditional powerlifting events (the other being the bench press). Deadlifts offer a change of pace from the squat, where you start fully loaded holding the bar. In a deadlift, you literally lift a very heavy weight off the ground. It doesn't get more basic than that!

> The 25 percent of your body that squats and deadlifts don't work is covered by the two core pressing movements: overhead press and bench press.

And for being so basic, it can be both brutal and also brutally effective. The deadlift is different from most lifts in that your body is unloaded when you begin the lift, meaning that you start from a dead stop, with no muscles engaged.

The squat works your entire lower body; the deadlift works the entire backside of your body. The two movements together represent nearly 75 percent of your musculature.

BARBELL OVERHEAD PRESS

The overhead press is just as it sounds—you press a weight over your head. In our case, we're talking about a barbell overhead press. Load a barbell with some weight, step up to it and press it over your head. Lower the weight in front of your face to shoulder height and press it over your head again. Very basic. Very effective.

BARBELL BENCH PRESS

Of all the exercises listed, none is as iconic as the bench press. "Dude, how much do you bench?" is a universal gym question when someone sees a big guy. And, if most people are going to do only one day a week in the gym, odds are the bench press is included in that day. Why? Because the bench pumps up the vanity muscles: chest and arms. Yeah, bulging chest and big guns are a great goal, but the bench press is only one part of a workout to build impressive muscle.

We can't stress this enough: Any weighted exercise can be extremely dangerous, but the bench press has most of 'em beat as the heavy weight is being suspended above your body. If your muscles fail or you make a mistake, there is a very real possibility of injury. A spotter should keep a close eye and two hands on the bar at all times while allowing you to do all the work. Spotters are extremely handy to assist in unracking and re-racking the weight to make sure it is secure.

If you can't find another human to act as your spotter, you can use a bench with spotter arms, perform your bench press inside a cage with safety arms set just a bit below your chest height or, as a last resort, use a Smith machine, a piece of equipment with a barbell fixed in its frame so the weight can only move up or down. Smith machines are safe, but don't really allow for a natural movement of the bar, and you can cheat by pushing a bit off-plane and the bar will still slide up. We recommend using very light weights without a spotter, and using a Smith machine when working with heavier weights safely.

Find the grip that works best for you; a standard grip will have your forearms at 90 degrees relative to your upper arms. The narrower your grip, the more you will work your triceps during the move, the wider the grip the more you will work your anterior deltoids. We recommend mixing in one wide grip (about 3 inches wider than standard grip) and one narrow grip (2–3 inches narrower than standard grip) per every two sets of a standard-grip bench press. Take note of where your hands are in relation to the smooth rings on the Olympic bar so you can repeat or vary your hand position from there.

When gripping the bar, slide your palm up behind the bar until your thumb touches underneath the bar. Grab the bar and rotate your hands back toward your toes so that your palm is under the bar. This rotation puts your hands, arms and shoulders in an optimal position for pressing the most weight.

TIP: Break the bar—grip the bar tightly, and mentally try and bend the bar until it breaks directly over your chest. Envision breaking a handful of spaghetti over boiling water (and try not to make yourself hungry—you have work to do!) and use that mental image to grip the bar strongly and break it in half from the second you grip the bar until you re-rack after your set.

Lifting Safely

You can very easily hurt yourself by exercising with weights. Well, duh. It is extremely easy to drop a weight or a bar on any exposed body part and cause some serious damage. Muscles fail, grips slip, people stumble with weights and the end result is a potentially very bad day for someone—don't let that be you.

If you're smart in the weight room, you can stay safe; always be familiar with the equipment you are using and never take it for granted that everything is in tip-top shape. Always check weight racks, benches and any equipment that you plan on using before you try to use it to lift any weight or protect you from keeping that weight off your body. Equipment wears out, so don't let a weak safety pin or missing bolt be the reason you get hurt when it's pretty easy to check before you start.

All the safety equipment in the gym isn't going to help you if you don't use it. Make sure safety bars are in place and engaged properly when you are using a cage, check the spotter pins and make sure any safety equipment is working properly before you add any weight.

Use a spotter, preferably one who understands proper form and is strong enough to help you if and when you need it. Always communicate with your spotter

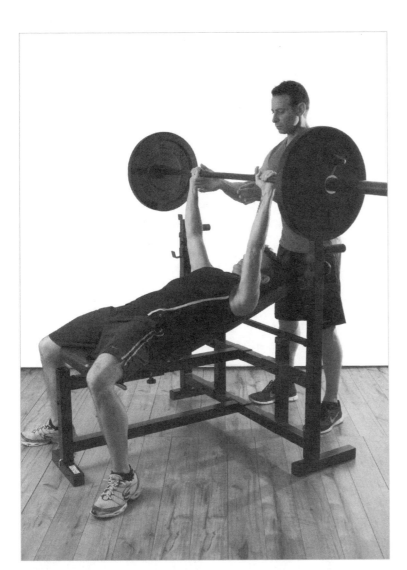

before and during the exercise (if you can). Verbalize how many reps you intend on completing so they know when to assist re-racking, and talk about a bail-out plan where they should lift or push the weights in an emergency.

Last, but in no way least, make sure you know what the hell you are doing before you add weight to any bar and put yourself underneath it. What you do in practice you will do when it counts, so make sure you know exactly what motion you will be using to raise, lower or lift weights safely. No spotter or safety equipment is going to bail you out if you're acting like a jackass with weights. If you don't know what you're doing then spend some time with a broomstick, length of PVC pipe or Olympic bar without any added weight.

Squat

PRIMARY MUSCLES: Quadriceps, gluteus maximus | SECONDARY MUSCLES: Hamstrings, hips, core

Work on achieving proper form by performing reps with a PVC pipe or a broomstick across your shoulders and a vertical mirror, partner or video camera aimed at your side. Check and adjust the alignment of your upper body, knees and hips before you get under the bar and add any weight at all.

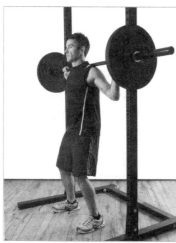

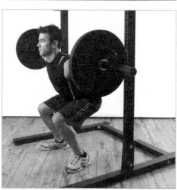

1 Place the bar in a stable, somewhat comfortable (see "Using a Pad" sidebar) position across your upper back at shoulder height. Stand centered under the bar and place your hands 6–8 inches wider than your shoulders on the bar in an overhand grip. Your knees should be slightly bent to allow you to get under the bar. Place your feet approximately shoulder-width apart and straighten your legs to lift the weight off the rack. Carefully step forward just enough to clear the bar of the J-cups. Stand up straight with your shoulders back (your chest should be as wide as possible) and keep your chin up, head looking straight ahead. Take a deep breath and tighten your abdominal muscles to stabilize your core and protect your back during the descent.

2 Rotate your hips backward and slowly descend as if you were about to sit down into a chair. Your knees should never extend farther than your toes and your shoulders, hips and ankles should form a straight line. Your weight should be resting just behind your midfoot, directly under your ankle bone. Do not let your knees bow in or you can cause some serious damage. If you cannot keep your knees in the proper line, you are trying to squat too much weight and are in danger of spraining or tearing your medial collateral ligament (MCL).

Continue descending in a controlled manner with your head and chest up until your thighs are parallel to the ground. Breathe out and drive your upper body straight up through your heels back to starting position. Do not bounce at the bottom or the top, and be extremely careful not to snap-lock and potentially hyperextend your knees at the top.

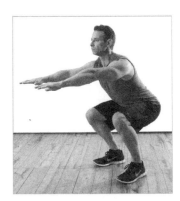

BODYWEIGHT VARIATION: To perform a basic unweighted squat—also called a "bodyweight squat"—stand up straight with shoulders back, chin up, head looking straight forward and a small, natural curve in your lower back. At no point during the movement should you hunch forward; your head and chest should remain "high" throughout the entire exercise. Your feet should be approximately shoulder-width apart and they can be rotated up to 45 degrees outward for comfort. Perform a squat as you would with a barbell, but raise your arms until they're parallel to the floor.

BOX SQUAT VARIATION: If you don't have a spotter or a rack with safety arms, box squats are a safe alternative to standard weighted squats. Position a stable object like a bench, a chair without arms, or a box behind you. If you start to lose your balance during the squat motion you can sit down to gain control. When performing the exercise, the downward motion should end when your glutes barely touch the bench, and then press through your heels back up to starting position.

USING A PAD

Some folks swear by it and there are even some really interesting variations of pads that clip onto the bar and look like something out of *Star Wars*. Pads can actually be responsible for more pain than a bare bar as they focus all of the bar's weight on your cervical vertebrae due to the added girth. A bare bar should actually not touch your spine at all, but rest on top of your trapezius muscle on either side of your neck. Also, pads can cause the weight to wobble or teeter-totter on your neck, and that's just a disaster waiting to happen all around. The bar should be stable on your back before you perform any movement. If you use a pad, make sure it is not adversely affecting the bar's position.

Front Squat

PRIMARY MUSCLES: Quadriceps | SECONDARY MUSCLES: Gluteus maximus

More work with less weight? Sign me up! Front squats are a great way to perform deeper, more intense squats with less weight than traditional back squats (page 108). Once you get the positioning right, they're also a bit more comfortable than an Olympic bar sitting across the top of your traps.

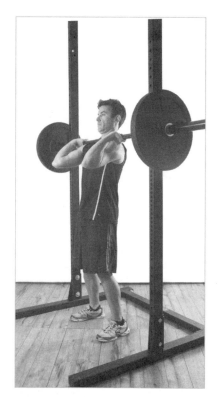

1 In a squat rack or cage, position an Olympic bar just below shoulder height. Step into the bar, positioning it on the natural shelf just above your chest and below your collarbone. Using your fingers (not your palms), hold the bar in position above your chest. Some people use three fingers, some use four. Your elbows should be pointing straight forward or slightly up, if possible. The bigger your biceps, the harder the positioning is. The higher you can get your elbows, the more stable you will be.

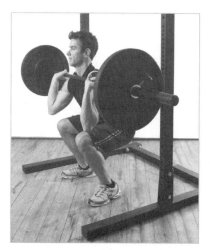

2 Lift the bar out of the rack and step back one step. Engage your core. Sit back slightly and lower your body in a typical squat. Your torso should be completely upright to support the bar on the front of your body rather than the back of your body. Core engagement is key.

Pause at the bottom, then push through your glutes and return to starting position.

Deadlift

PRIMARY MUSCLES: Hamstrings, gluteus maximus, lower back | SECONDARY MUSCLES: Hips, trapezius

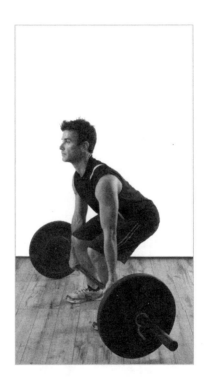 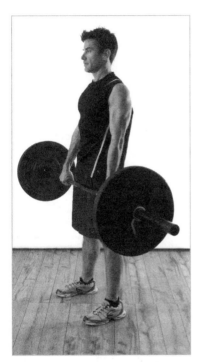

1 Starting with an Olympic bar on the floor, choose a light weight and place an equal number and weight of plates on either end. Position your feet shoulder-width apart with your toes under the bar and your shins very close to the bar. Grasp the bar with either an overhand or mixed grip (one underhand, one overhand) a few inches outside of your legs in relation to the bar. Push your hips directly back slightly, lift your chest and keep your chin up with your head looking directly in front of you. Do not hunch your shoulders, or lean forward; your back should be primarily straight with a natural curve.

2 Take a deep breath, and then drive through your heels and extend your legs to lift the bar straight up toward the top of your thighs while rising to a standing position. Finish the move by pressing your hips forward, aligning your shoulders, hips, knees and ankles in a straight line. Do not lean back at the top of the movement, this will put undue stress on your lower back.

Slowly and carefully reverse the move to lower the bar to the floor. Do not bend over and place the bar on the ground—the bar should follow the exact same path as it did while you were raising it. Do not drop the bar from the top or you'll be missing out on half of the exercise!

Overhead Press

PRIMARY MUSCLES: Shoulders | SECONDARY MUSCLES: Triceps

The one exercise that's most often overlooked as a powerful mass-gainer is the simple overhead press. This extremely beneficial movement actually engages all the major muscle groups in your body and helps to build a strong core and massive upper body. It's sometimes a little disconcerting to press heavy weights over your head, but this move is extremely effective and is very safe when you use the right technique and the proper weights. Start light—a broomstick, PVC pipe or unweighted bar should be all you use until you have mastered the technique.

1 The bar should be positioned on a squat rack at shoulder height. It is recommended that you practice this exercise with no weight until you are familiar with the proper form. Grip the bar with an overhand grip just outside your shoulders. Rotate your elbows so they are under the bar, pointing directly away from your torso. Raise your chest and keep your head looking straight forward. You will need to tilt your head back a little bit so the bar can clear your chin when you press the bar up. Unrack the bar and take a small step backward so the bar can clear the rack when you press it. Your feet should be even with each other and shoulder-width apart.

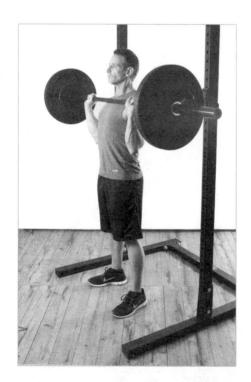

TIP: Squeeze your glutes, tighten your core and rotate your hips forward to "tuck" your tailbone between your legs. You should not have a large arch in your lower back; this will cause excess pressure on your lower back, leading to pain and possible injury. Fix your form and lighten your weight—or both—in order to perform this exercise properly to reap the maximum muscle- and strength-building benefits.

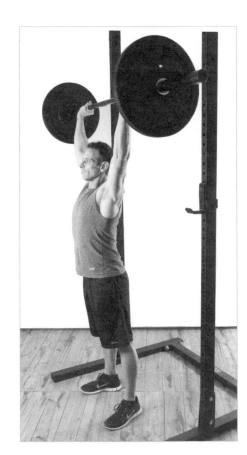

2 Take a deep breath, squeeze your glutes and core, and tuck your tailbone to provide a strong, stable base. Press the bar in a straight line directly overhead. Once the bar has passed the top of your head, press your upper body and head forward so the bar is directly overhead and the inside of your elbows are about laterally even with your ears. When the bar reaches its apex, your entire body should be in a strong, stable position; your legs, glutes, core, shoulders, upper back and arms should all be activated to keep the weight in place.

Slowly lower the bar, tilting your head back and controlling the bar's descent until it softly touches your collarbone. (Softly! Your collarbone, or clavicle, can be broken by less than 10 pounds of force!) Exhale.

DUMBBELL VARIATION: This exercise can be done with dumbbells instead of an Olympic bar, following the same instructions as with the barbell. Dumbbells allow you to use lighter weights and the independent arm motion also strengthens the supporting muscles.

PUSH PRESS VARIATION: If you need a little help starting the upward press, you can use a bit of leg drive to start the motion. Commonly referred to as a "Push Press," this movement is when you push up with your legs to initiate pressing the dumbbells or barbell overhead. A slight squat straight down and rapid extension upward will help get the bar moving and help you through a sticking point. This is a small movement, not a deep squat and explosion like you would use to perform squat thrusters.

Flat Bench Press

PRIMARY MUSCLES: Chest | SECONDARY MUSCLES: Shoulders, triceps

Flat, Incline and Decline Bench Press exercises are far from simple to perform properly; they are much more complicated than lying on a bench and pushing a weight up, as developing perfect form will enable you to lift more weight more often and to build a bigger, stronger chest. Start with a broomstick or unweighted Olympic bar and practice proper technique throughout the entire movement before you add any weight at all. Oh, and find a spotter. Really.

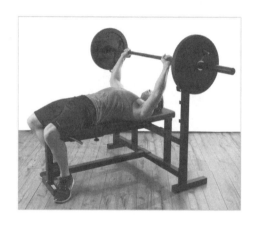

1 Check the bar position on the rack. When you lie under the bar you should be able to extend your elbows completely when you lift the bar off the safety pegs. You should never be raising the bar and moving it forward away from the safety supports with bent elbows.

Lie back on the bench with your feet flat on the floor as wide as you comfortably can. Your heels should be solidly planted and very stable. If your legs are too short to be securely flat on the floor, slide a couple of 45-pound plates under your feet.

Squeeze your shoulder blades together and broaden your chest. This will lift your lower back off the bench such that your glutes, shoulder blades and head are touching the bench. Along with your feet on the floor, your position on the bench needs to be stable; this is why it is important to practice this positioning without weight!

Position yourself on the bench so that there is enough room for you to press the bar straight up from your chest without hitting the safety pins (or rack or J-cups) when you push the weight up. You also do not want to be so far away from the supports that you are in a weak arm position when you unrack the bar. Since each bench is different, test out your position by using an unweighted bar for warm-ups.

Grip the bar tightly with your desired hand position as described in the grip method on page 129. Tuck your elbows toward your sides and keep them as close to your body as you can during the entire movement.

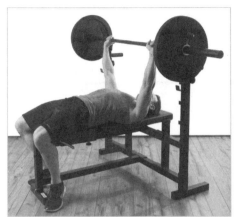 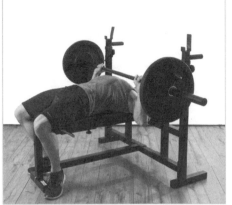 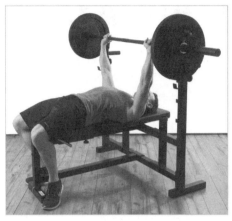

2 Press the bar straight up off the safety pins and extend your elbows into a locked position before moving the weight directly over your sternum. Do not unrack and descend the bar in one movement; the lateral momentum and possible overcompensation can cause the bar to fall on your ribcage or toward your neck or head. Be extremely careful and deliberate when you unrack the weight; extend your arms and get the bar on the right plane straight up, about 1–2 inches below your nipples or even with the bottom of your sternum.

3 Inhale, and in a controlled manner, lower the bar until it touches your chest.

4 Press the bar directly up in a straight line back to starting position using your chest, arms and even the heels of your feet. Keep your glutes on the bench, shoulder blades retracted and chest up throughout the entire fluid movement as you breathe out. Extend your arms fully such that your elbows are straight and the weight is stable above you.

TIP: Press, don't row. Sometimes you'll get in a rhythm when pressing too fast, and the top and bottom of the movement will have a bit of a circular motion. This robs you of power and saps your strength because you have to continually pull the bar back into position to press. In a worst-case scenario, you can lose control of the bar. Your bench press should be like a piston, a powerful move straight up and a controlled stroke straight down.

Incline Bench Press

PRIMARY MUSCLES: Upper chest | SECONDARY MUSCLES: Shoulders, triceps

Incline bench press is harder for most people than the flat bench and will usually require you to use less weight. Most of the setup is similar, yet the motion is slightly different and requires practice to nail proper form. This exercise targets the upper pecs more so than the flat bench does and helps to yield a thicker, stronger chest. Play with hand position on the bar to see what feels comfortable to you. Also, changing hand placement is a great way to stress the chest in new and interesting ways.

1 Set the bench angle between 20 and 40 degrees. The steeper the angle (or the higher the head portion of the bench), the more you will be activating your shoulder muscles while using less of your chest.

Sit on the seat area of the bench and place both feet firmly on the ground on either side of the bench to form a stable, wide stance. Lie back on the bench and squeeze your shoulder blades together as you did in the flat bench. Grip the bar as described in the flat bench press example, and tuck your elbows in. Keep them as close to your sides as possible throughout the movement. Breathe in, extend your elbows and press the bar straight up from the safety pegs. Carefully bring the bar directly over your upper chest and pause.

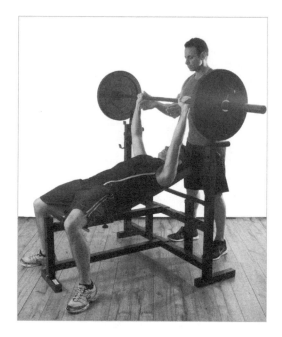

TIP: Your elbows should be tucked in close to your torso more than during the flat bench press due to the change in the push plane of the bar. For incline, you will be lowering the bar and pressing from the top of your sternum, and to de-stress your shoulders, your elbows should be at 45 degrees on both sides in relation to your torso.

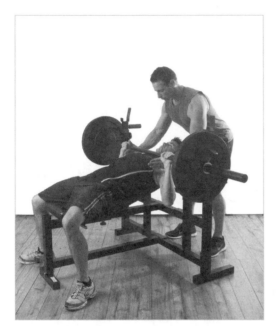 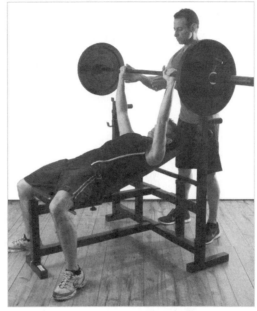

2 Descend in a controlled manner until the bar touches your chest at the top of your sternum.

3 Exhale and drive the bar straight up using your chest, arms, delts and even your feet. Extend your elbows straight into a stable position (some call it a locked position, some say it's semi-locked—as long as you don't snap your elbows straight and hyperextend them you should be A-OK). The point is to keep the weight stable before your next rep.

Dip

PRIMARY MUSCLES: Triceps **|** SECONDARY MUSCLES: Chest, shoulders

Your angle and how wide the bars on your dip station are will dictate how much the various muscles are involved. A closer grip is more triceps, wider is more shoulders (not ideal). A more forward lean means more chest is involved. Try to stay as upright as possible with your elbows as close to your body as you can manage.

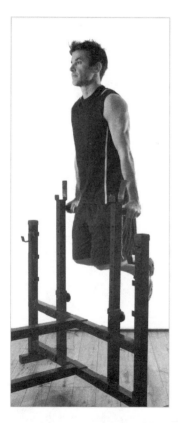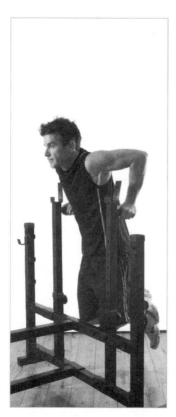

1 Step between two dip bars that are about shoulder-width apart. Non-parallel bars allow you to find a hand position (rotated in or out) and a width that is more comfortable. Grip the top of the bars securely and extend your arms completely with your body leaning about 5 degrees forward.

2 Lower your body in a controlled manner by bending your arms at the elbows. Be cautious of elbow or shoulder pain and adjust your positioning to lessen any strain. When your upper arms and forearms are roughly 90 degrees in relation to each other, your upper arms are parallel to the dip bar or your feel a deep stretch in your chest or shoulders, pause your descent.

Drive your hands back down toward your knees by using your triceps to return your arms to a fully extended position.

Triceps Pressdown

PRIMARY MUSCLES: Triceps | **SECONDARY MUSCLES:** Core

Most people think massive arms come from just building the biggest biceps possible, but developing defined triceps will not only emphasize upper arm mass but triceps strength will also promote more balanced musculature and help prevent overuse injuries. The Triceps Pressdown is extremely beneficial for building stronger, more defined triceps and more complete upper arm strength.

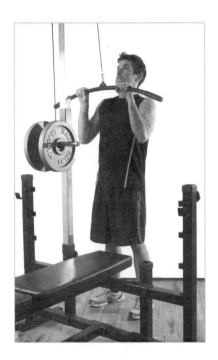
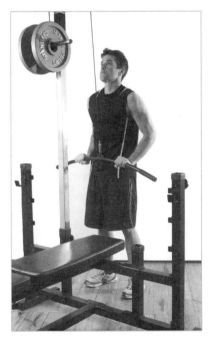

1 Using a triceps pressdown machine or lat pulldown machine, grasp the bar with an overhand grip (palms toward the ground). Pull the bar down until your elbows are aligned with the outside of your body; both will be bent and the bar will be about chin height in front of your body. Engage your core.

2 Keeping your elbows in place, use your triceps (not your shoulders) to pull the bar down in an arc toward your hips. Squeeze your triceps to keep the bar in position, and hold for 1–3 seconds. Do not hunch forward; keep your core engaged and back straight throughout the entire movement.

Slowly return the bar to starting position at your chin.

Leg Press

PRIMARY MUSCLES: Quadriceps | SECONDARY MUSCLES: Hamstrings, gluteus maximus

A distant second to the squat, the leg press still an overall good mass builder in the legs. Where it hits your muscles greatly depends on the machine and where you place your feet, including foot angle and depth. Play with foot positioning using low weights to get a feel for what is comfortable for you. Feet higher up on the platform will focus on the hamstrings more, lower works the quads. You'll also notice different muscles being activated when you take your feet wider or narrower. NOTE: When using ANY machine, check the instructions and manufacturer's warning labels and perform the exercise according to their recommendations. Each machine is different, and the description below is just a general overview.

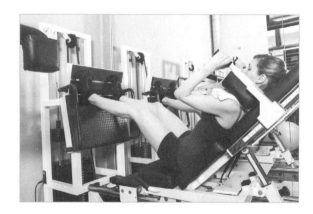

1 Sit in a 45-degree leg press machine. Position your feet so your knees are over your toes. Your feet should be pointed slightly outward and shoulder-width apart.

2 Push through your heels and fully extend your legs.

Pause, then SLOWLY lower the weight to the starting position.

Hamstring Curl

PRIMARY MUSCLES: Hamstrings | SECONDARY MUSCLES: Gluteus maximus

Full range of motion is important. If you aren't squeezing your butt at the end of the rep, you aren't doing a full rep. Lower the weight and start over to make sure you get a full rep. Don't bounce the weights. If you aren't feeling it in your hamstrings and glutes when you're done, your form needs work. NOTE: When using ANY machine, check the instructions and manufacturer's warning labels and perform the exercise according to their recommendations. Each machine is different, and the description below is just a general overview.

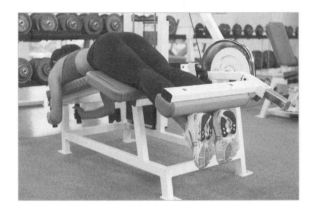

1 Lie face down on a leg curl machine. Position both feet with toes pointing slightly outward.

2 Contract your hamstrings and glutes to bring your heels to your glutes.

Pause, then return to starting position.

Barbell Row

PRIMARY MUSCLES: Latissimus dorsi | SECONDARY MUSCLES: Back

To get the most out of this lift, squeeze your shoulder blades together and bring your elbows to the ceiling and you'll feel it where you're supposed to: across the broad muscles in your upper back.

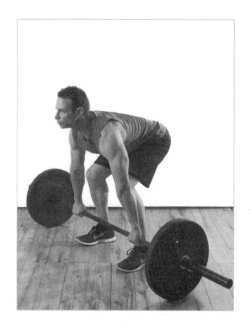

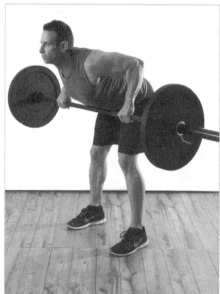

1 Place a barbell on the floor and position yourself over it. With your knees slightly bent and your back straight, bend forward at the waist until your back is approximately parallel with the ground. Reach down and grasp the barbell with an overhand grip and arms fully extended.

2 Using primarily your upper back, not your arms, pull the bar to your waist or lower torso. To activate your back more than your arms, mentally focus on squeezing your back and shoulder blades together as tightly as possible. You will naturally use some arms, but the key is to minimize their involvement!

Pause, then return to starting position with your arms fully extended.

Low Bar Row

PRIMARY MUSCLES: Latissimus dorsi, upper back | SECONDARY MUSCLES: Arms, core

This upper back exercise allows you to target the latissimus dorsi with an upward rowing motion. This changes the plane of resistance up from the bent-over rows and allows you to perform more back-strengthening exercises in a set. Watch your grip. A narrow grip will limit your range of motion, as your wrists will hit your chest before you have finished the move; too wide of a grip will place unnecessary stress on your shoulders.

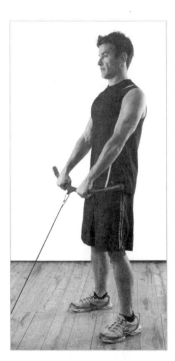 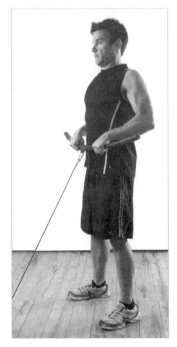

1 Affix a flat or lat bar to a low pulley and adjust the weights to allow for completion of your set. Grasp the bar with both hands approximately shoulder-width apart, depending on the length of the bar. Step back far enough to remove any slack from the cable and stand in an athletic position with back bent naturally, knees slightly bent and feet approximately shoulder-width apart.

2 Using the large muscles of your upper back, pull the weight up toward your chest, keeping your elbows parallel with the cable. Squeeze your shoulder blades together as the bar nears your chest. Pause.

Lower slowly back to starting position.

Dumbbell Shrug

PRIMARY MUSCLES: Trapezius | SECONDARY MUSCLES: Shoulders

This can be done with either a barbell or dumbbells. Dumbbells tend to offer a greater range of motion but also more propensity for cheating. With either dumbbells or barbells, focus on the squeeze at the top and slowly, we repeat slowly, descend the weight. Shrugs should NOT be pulling your shoulders to your ears. Instead, lean forward a bit, pull through your traps and back and pause at the top. This is crucial.

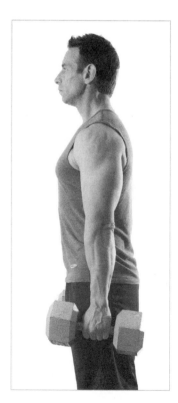
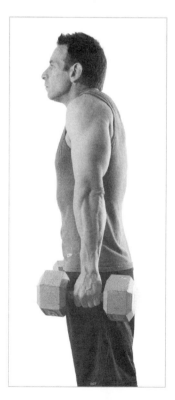

1 Grasp two dumbbells of the same weight. Hold them by your sides with your shoulders relaxed. Lean forward at the hips a bit, letting the weights hang just in front of you.

2 Flex your traps and pull your shoulders through your back. In other words, shrug. Pause at the top, then slowly lower to the starting position, but never fully relax your shoulders.

BARBELL VARIATION: This exercise can also be performed with a barbell. In a squat rack or cage, place a barbell at about mid-thigh height on supporting bars. If you do not have a rack, begin the movement by performing a deadlift (see page 111 for description). Grasp the barbell using an overhand grip (palms toward your body) with your hands just outside the width of your hips, keeping both knees slightly bent. Engage your core to stabilize your back, and straighten your knees and stand fully upright to lift the bar off the rack; do not lock out your knees. Continue to engage your core and pull upward through your traps, shoulders and upper back to lift the bar. Your shoulders should raise toward your ears. Squeeze your trapezius muscles at the top and hold the upper position for 1–3 seconds. Slowly return to starting position.

Barbell Curl

PRIMARY MUSCLES: Biceps | SECONDARY MUSCLES: Forearms

This can be done with either a straight bar or an EZ curl bar. If you vary your hand position on the EZ bar, you can target different areas of the biceps and work the entire muscle. Focus on keeping your elbows steady and static, lifting the weight consciously with your biceps, not your shoulders. There is a great tendency to bounce the weight. Resist this urge at all costs.

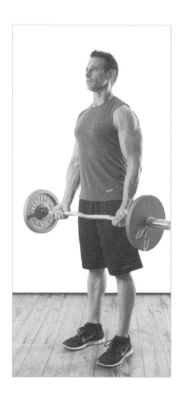

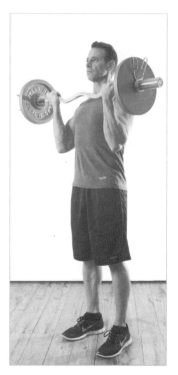

1 Grasp a barbell with an underhand grip. Lock your elbows either in place or to your hips/sides.

2 Raise the bar in an arc toward your shoulders, never fully reaching your shoulders. You want to stop when the biceps aren't doing the work anymore; the shoulders take over near the peak, and you want to keep the biceps engaged throughout the movement.

Pause, then slowly lower the bar to starting position.

VARIATION: This exercise can also be performed with dumbbells.

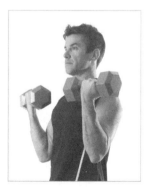

Hammer Curl

PRIMARY MUSCLES: Biceps | SECONDARY MUSCLES: Forearms

In order to build bigger biceps, you need to target the muscles from multiple angles. The palm-inward grip of the hammer curl is one such variation that helps to work the forearms as well.

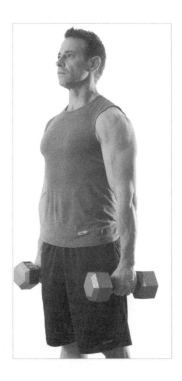
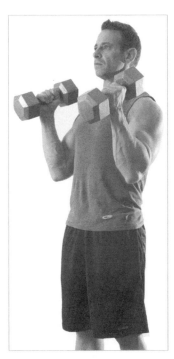

1 Squat straight down and grasp two dumbbells. Lift them to the outside of both hips, palms toward your body. Engage your core.

2 Using your biceps (not your shoulders), lift the weights toward your shoulders, hinging at the elbows and keeping both elbows as close to the sides of your torso as possible. The heads of the dumbbells should travel straight to your shoulders, stopping just short of touching. (Your arms and the weight should look like a hammer). Squeeze both biceps at the top, pause for 1–3 seconds. Return to starting position, pausing at the bottom.

1-Arm Dumbbell Row

PRIMARY MUSCLES: Latissimus dorsi | SECONDARY
MUSCLES: Biceps

This should be done with the strictest of form until you have mastered the exercise. Be sure to focus on pulling up with your back muscles and driving your elbow toward the ceiling rather than pulling the weight with your biceps.

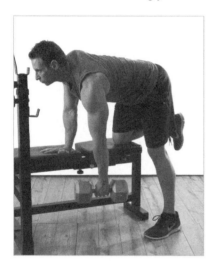
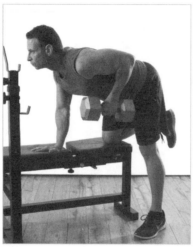

1 Position yourself on a flat bench with your left knee and left hand on the bench for support. Place your right leg slightly back on the ground for support. Grasp a dumbbell with your right hand directly beneath your right shoulder.

2 Pull the dumbbell to your side until it makes contact with your waist. Pause, then return to starting position. Don't put the dumbbell back on the ground.

Continue until all reps are complete, then repeat on your left side.

Close-Grip Bench Press

PRIMARY MUSCLES: Triceps | SECONDARY
MUSCLES: Chest, shoulders

Play with hand position quite a bit on this exercise to find out what's comfortable and doesn't aggravate your elbows, shoulders and wrists. This is also a great lift to do with an EZ curl bar.

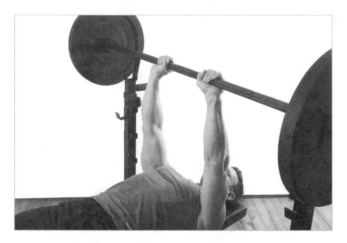

1 Position yourself on a flat bench as you would for a standard Flat Bench Press (page 114). Grasp the bar with your hands just inside shoulder-width. Dismount the bar and hold at the top, arms fully extended.

2 Lower the bar until your hands or bar touches your chest. Pause, then push the bar away from your chest, returning to your starting position.

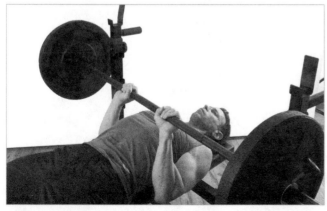

Shoulder Raise   PRIMARY MUSCLES: Shoulders

Shoulder raises should be done both to the sides and to the front. We recommend one full set to the sides followed by one full set to the front. Do not go heavy, but instead use lighter weights and slow, controlled motions. If the weight doesn't feel heavy enough at the start, it should after 10 or 12 reps. Pause for a second at the top for extra effect. These are awesome to use Rest-Pause style.

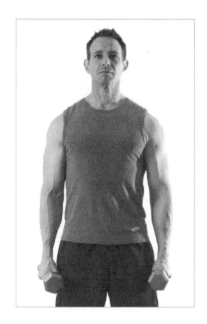

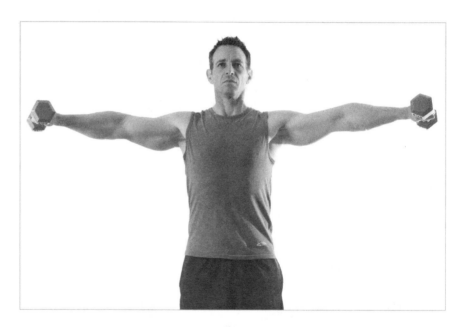

1 Grasp two dumbbells at your sides using an overhand grip, with the insides of your fists facing your body and thumbs roughly adjacent to your upper thighs.

2 Raise them away from your body to the sides and pause for 1–3 seconds when the weights are level with your shoulders. Then lower slowly to your sides. Repeat until you've completed half of the given reps for a workout before moving on to step 3.

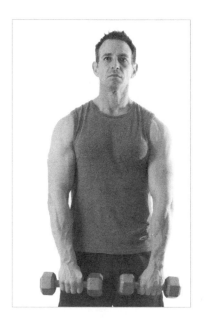
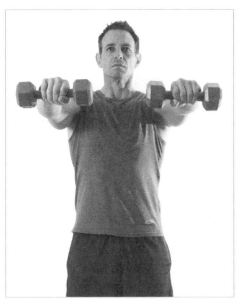

3 Bring the dumbbells around toward the front of your body, with your palms facing the fronts of your hips. Your elbows should be slightly bent, core engaged to keep your back straight, knees slightly bent in an athletic posture.

4 Raise your arms directly in front of your body until the weights are at shoulder level. Your arms should be straight but your elbows not in a fully locked-out position. Pause for 1–3 seconds, then lower slowly back to starting position.

Repeat steps 3–4 for the remainder of the required reps for a workout.

Calf Raise

PRIMARY MUSCLES: Calves | SECONDARY MUSCLES: Core

Foot position plays a large role in which muscles of the calf get worked in this exercise, and you will need to experiment with it based on which area of the calf you would like to work that day.

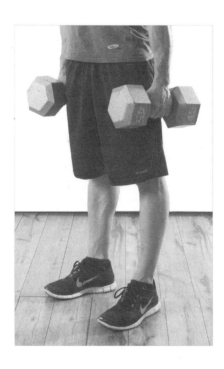
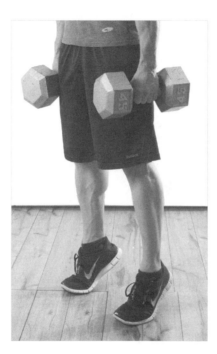

1 Holding a barbell or two dumbbells, lift the weight toward your waist and hold with your arms fully extended.

2 With your legs approximately shoulder-width apart and your toes pointed forward, press through the balls of your feet and raise your entire body and weight straight up. Maintain your balance on the balls of your feet and squeeze your calves to hold the "up" position for 1–3 seconds.

Slowly lower your heels back down to the floor.

Romanian Deadlift (RDL)

PRIMARY MUSCLES: Hamstrings | SECONDARY MUSCLES: Gluteus maximus

This is probably THE BEST hamstring builder out there. I love these. They're just fun. Squeezing the glutes on the lockout at the top of the lift is key.

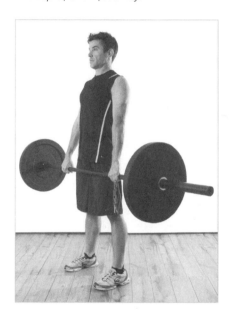

1 Grasping a barbell with an overhand grip, stand upright with the barbell at leg level, arms fully extended. Keep the core, lower back, glutes and hips tight and focused.

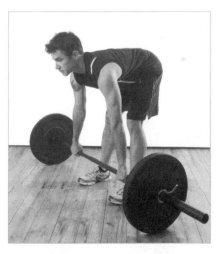

2 Never relaxing the core, lower back, glutes or hips, slowly lower the bar toward the ground, not quite touching the ground

Pause, then return to starting position.

Hip Raise

PRIMARY MUSCLES: Hips | SECONDARY MUSCLES: Gluteus maximus, core

Along with the Weighted Hip Thrust (page 135), this is a fantastic exercise for overall core strength while focusing on your often overlooked and underappreciated hips and glutes. The longer you hold and squeeze at the top, the more this works your glutes, abs and lower back. The more often you raise and descend, the more you concentrate the strengthening of your hips.

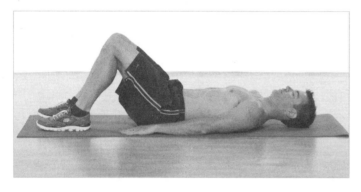

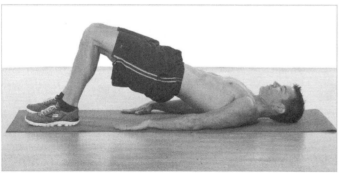

1 Lie flat on your back with your feet flat on the floor and knees bent so that your lower legs are perpendicular to floor. Your arms should be extended alongside your body with your palms down.

2 Pressing your heels into the floor, contract your abs and raise your glutes off the floor. Bring your pelvis toward the ceiling until your body forms a straight line from your sternum to your knees. Your upper back, head, arms and feet should all remain in contact with the ground. Squeeze your abs, brace your lower back and contract your glutes to maintain a "bridge" position for 5–30 seconds. Reverse the motion and slowly bring your butt back toward the floor.

Weighted Hip Thrust

PRIMARY MUSCLES: Hips, gluteus maximus, hamstrings | SECONDARY MUSCLES: Lower back, lower abs

Hip raises are a runner or triathlete's secret weapon. Too often during cycling and running, the weakest muscles are in a multisport athlete's lower back and hips, and they fatigue more quickly than the larger quads and hamstrings. Any athlete is only as strong as their weakest muscle groups, and hip raises can help strengthen those problem areas—all in one move!

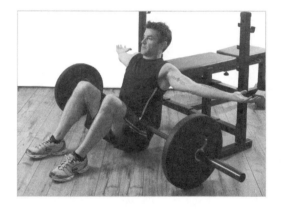

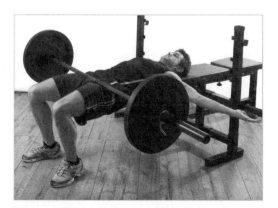

1 Sit on the floor and position a bench behind your upper back so that your shoulder blades make contact with the edge of the bench. Place your feet flat on the floor and lay a weighted bar, medicine ball or weight plate across your hips or at the very top of your pelvis (make sure the weight doesn't roll or shift to hit you in the genitals). Extend your arms out to your sides, parallel to the floor, or rest them on your chest.

2 Driving through your heels, use your hamstrings, hips and glutes to raise your pelvis toward the ceiling and slide your upper back onto the bench. Your body should form a straight line from head to knees. Squeeze your abs and glutes, and brace your lower back to hold the flat position for 3–5 seconds. In a slow and controlled manner, lower your butt back to the ground, carefully sliding your upper back off the bench.

TIP: Once you perfect your form, you can perform this movement as an explosive exercise. Just make sure that you do not hyperextend your back at the top or hit your tailbone on the floor at the bottom. Of course, it is imperative that you make sure the weight is light enough for you to handle and does not shift during the move. Be smart, be safe and choose your weights accordingly.

Landmine

PRIMARY MUSCLES: Abdominals, obliques | SECONDARY MUSCLES: Arms, shoulders, hips, gluteus maximus, lower back

This dynamic ab exercise works the entire core. Depending on the weight, it can be extremely physically taxing. Approach this movement with respect and humility.

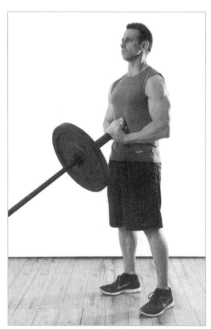
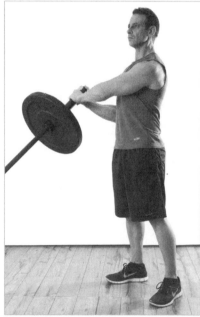

1 Place a 45-pound plate flat on the floor and position one end of a full-size Olympic bar in the plate's center hole on a 45-degree angle so that the tip of the bar is held in place, or in the corner of a room so the bar doesn't slide or roll away from you. Place both hands on the opposite end of the bar and raise it to chest height. The bar should be diagonal to your body, pointed away from your torso directly in front of you. Your feet should be shoulder-width apart, knees slightly bent, head up and shoulders back in an athletic stance.

2 In an arcing motion, brace your core and bring the bar to the right side of your body without twisting your hips. Your shoulders should remain in line with your hips, pointed straight ahead as in the starting position. Hold this position with your core flexed for 3–5 seconds. Return to starting position by swinging the bar in a reverse arc.

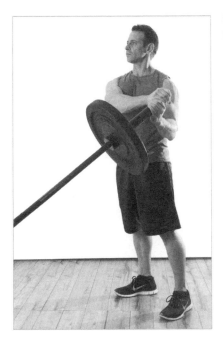

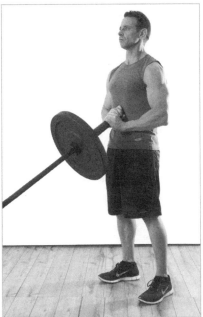

3 Repeat to the left side using the opposite motion.

4 After returning to the top position, bring the bar down toward your waist, pause for 3–5 seconds and press back up to the top position.

TIP: You can add weight to the end of the bar nearest your hands to make this a much more challenging move. We recommend starting with just the bar and then adding weight slowly. The more weight you have, the harder it is to stop the bar's momentum at the end of each arc, and the more it will work your opposing oblique muscles to keep your torso straight.

Bird Dog

PRIMARY MUSCLES: Gluteus maximus | SECONDARY MUSCLES: Hamstrings, deltoids, hips, abdominals

This is a very good low-stress glute exercise. If you can't do hip raises or weighted hip thrusts for any reason, these are a good alternative. Treat them as a progression to get you to hip thrusts, which are overall a better glute exercise, though more physically demanding. The effectiveness of this move is about how much you squeeze your core and glutes. If you half-ass it (pun intended), this is just a pretty boring waste of time.

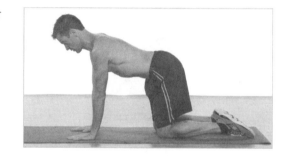

1 Get on your hands and knees with your legs bent 90 degrees, knees under your hips, toes on the floor and hands on the floor directly below your shoulders. Keep your head and spine neutral; do not let your head lift or sag. Contract your abdominal muscles to prevent your back from sagging; keep your back flat from shoulders to butt for the entire exercise.

2 In one slow and controlled motion, simultaneously raise your right leg and left arm until they're on the same flat plane as your back. Your leg should be parallel to the ground, not raised above your hip; your arm should extend directly out from your shoulder and your biceps should be level with your ear. Hold this position for 3–5 seconds and then slowly lower your arm and leg back to starting position.

That's 1 rep. Switch sides and repeat.

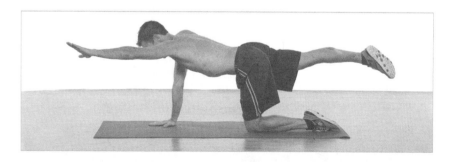

TIP: If you want to kick it up a notch, add a light dumbbell to your hand to work your delts and force your core to stabilize more. You can even add an ankle weight to work your hamstrings and glutes.

Plank

PRIMARY MUSCLES: Abdominals | SECONDARY MUSCLES: Gluteus maximus, lower back

Plank has replaced crunches as the "go to" ab exercise for fashionable fitness magazines...and here as well! It has many variants for progression as you advance: you can perform with your feet elevated on a bench, a BOSU Balance Trainer, suspended in a hanging exercise band and more.

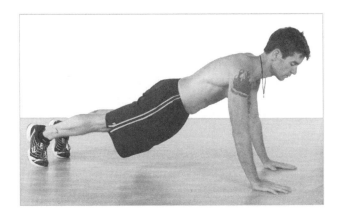

THE POSITION: Place your hands on the ground approximately shoulder-width apart, making sure your fingers point straight ahead and your arms are straight but your elbows not locked. Step your feet back until your body forms a straight line from head to feet. Your feet should be about 6 inches apart with the weight in the balls of your feet. Engage your core to keep your spine from sagging; don't sink into your shoulders.

Wood Chop

PRIMARY MUSCLES: Abdominals, obliques | SECONDARY MUSCLES: Gluteus maximus, hamstrings, arms, shoulders, upper back

Slightly different than the traditional wood chop, this is an overall body and core workout, while the cable version is a pure core exercise. For maximal abdominal activation, when you raise the weight above your head, hold it there and squeeze your abs as if you're about to take a punch.

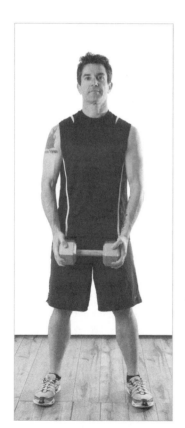

1 Grasp a dumbbell, plate or kettlebell with both hands and stand up straight in an "athletic stance": shoulders back, head high, back straight, hands at sides, knees with a slight bend, feet about shoulder-width apart with toes pointed slightly outward.

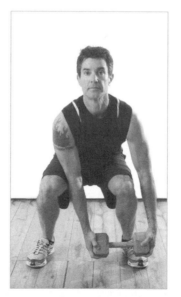

2 With your weight in your heels, initiate a squat (see page 108 for proper squat technique) and drop your torso straight down until your legs are past parallel; your butt should be as close to the floor as you can get without falling backward. Do not let your knees bow inward, which can cause injury. Slowly bring the weight toward your left foot using your arms; your shoulders and hips should remain pointing straight forward. Do not lean to the left because the imbalance of the weight helps to work your right obliques to maintain proper position.

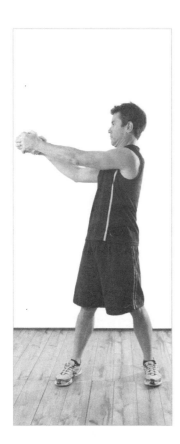
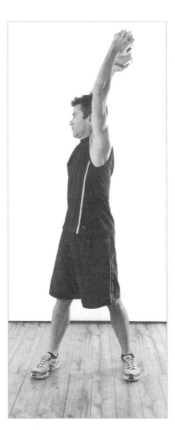

3 Pressing through your heels, raise your torso straight up and lift the weight up and toward the right side of your body.

4 When the weight reaches your right shoulder, twist your core to the right, continue raising the weight and press it directly overhead, with both arms fully extended, back straight, head up high and looking to the right. Your entire core should be engaged to keep you in a stable position, with abs and glutes contracted. Your hips should be pointing forward as much as possible; you are rotating with your obliques and torso, not your hips. Of course, there will be some hip rotation, but keep it to a minimum.

Slowly return the weight back to starting position in a controlled manner. Repeat to the left side. That's 1 rep.

TIP: Do not twist in the first position to bring the weight to one foot or the other. Drop straight down into your deep squat and slightly rotate your arms—not your hips or shoulders—to bring the weight into the down position.

Next Steps

We've talked about *7 Weeks to Getting Ripped* quite a bit throughout this book, and as our best-seller to date, it's really the fitness program that put us on the map. Tens of thousands of copies and about a million visits to www.7weekstofitness.com later, we know it's a program that has helped a lot of people out on their fitness journey. The full-body program was designed to be a cornerstone of developing strength, athletic ability and sculpting a lean physique.

When we created the program for this book, our plan was to develop a muscle-building program to use during an "off-season" from athletic activity and use *Getting Ripped* or one of our other bodyweight programs or challenges during the rest of a six-month cycle. By the time we were done with it, we had different ideas what an "off-season" really was!

JASON: I like to alternate between training for strength, size and athletic ability throughout a six-month cycle. My six-month rotation is much more weight-intensive than Brett's:

2 months: Comprehensive strength training

2 months: *7 Weeks to 10 Pounds of Muscle*

2 months: *7 Weeks to Getting Ripped*

In between each program, I'll take a few days off and then test myself with some challenge like 1,000 push-ups, 100 pull-ups and 300 sit-ups in a day, or test out my max squat or deadlift. Those little challenges and goals help me keep pushing myself through each program and continually work on improving my max.

BRETT: Unlike Jason, I like to run. A lot. While I can't lift anything near what he can in the weight department, he's not too keen on logging 50- to 100-mile weeks while training for a marathon or ultra. For me, *Getting Ripped* is my go-to program nearly year-round, and I constantly test the new programs for every one of our fitness books: *Ultimate Obstacle Race Training*, *7 Weeks to a Triathlon* and more. *7 Weeks to 10 Pounds of Muscle* forces me to cut out a majority of my running and is therefore my July/August "off-season" tool for rebuilding my body and adding back some muscle after spending the other 10 months of the year trying to be as light and strong as possible. Why July and August? I live in Phoenix, and it's hotter than the surface of the sun those two months, so due to that there are very few triathlons and marathons held then.

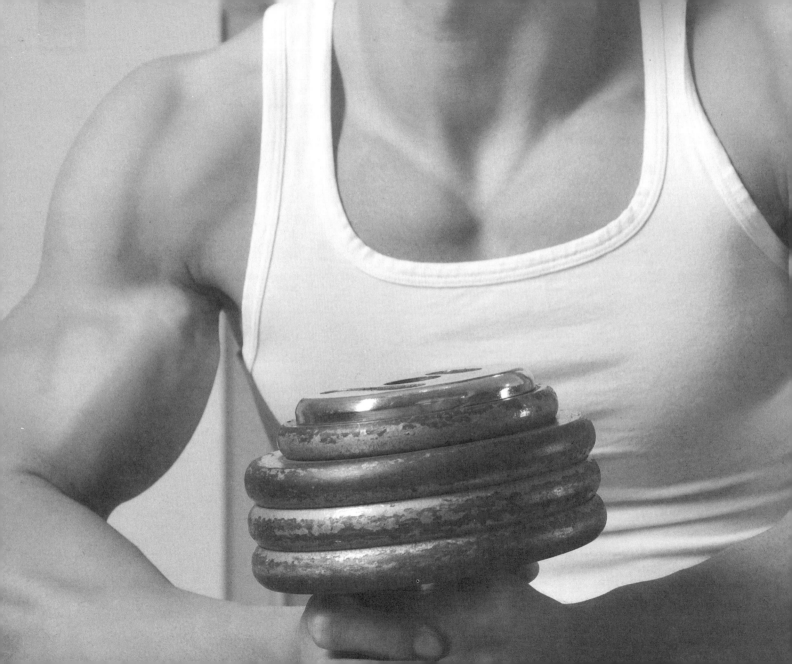

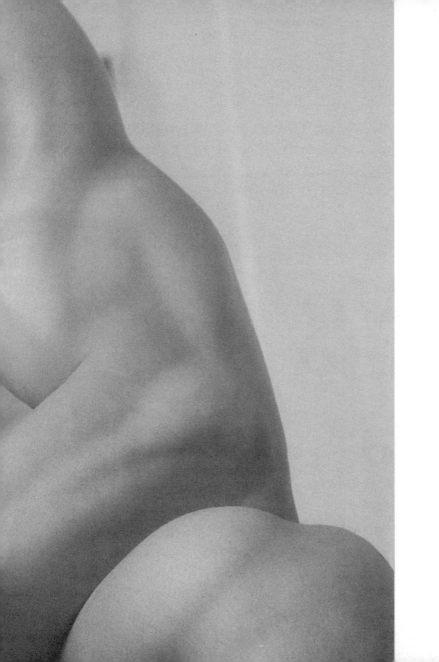

IAPPENDIX

Warming Up & Stretching

Prior to your workout, you want to warm up and loosen any tight muscles—but not put them through any rigorous stretching as that can wreak havoc on cold, inflexible muscle fibers. Stretches are to be performed only on warm muscles, optimally after you've completed your workout, in order to promote blood flow and speed up healing (and growing). A good stretch is one where you extend the muscle and work it through a full range of motion, and the stretch should be a slow and controlled movement—never bounce!

Here's the proper progression to keep in mind:

1. **Basic Warm-Up:** Walk, jog, jumping jacks—raise your heart rate slightly, loosen up stiff muscles).

2. **Dynamic Warm-Up/Shake Out:** After at least 5 minutes of warm-up, shake out your arms and legs and perform some of the dynamic warm-ups listed on page 149. Focus on the moves relating to the part of your body that you'll be working first. You can come back to the dynamic warm-ups before you start to work the other part of your body.

3. **Perform Bodyweight (or Lightweight) Exercises:** Focusing on maintaining perfect form, perform 10–12 lightweight or bodyweight reps of each major exercise before you choose the appropriate weight for your workout.

4. **Work Out:** Be mindful of your form on every rep. Maintain your intensity and crush your workout.

5. **Shake Out/Stretch:** Shake out your tight muscles, then perform some stretches listed on page 151.

6. **Eat:** Immediately post-workout, start eating. See page 86.

7. **Rest:** Jump-start the building process by resting. A 20-minute nap after eating never hurts.

Basic Warm-Up: Raise Your Heart Rate & Limber Up: No matter the workout, we recommend spending 5–10 minutes on a treadmill, stationary bike or rowing machine just to get the blood pumping, muscles warmed up and joints lubricated. There's no need to exert yourself, but just get everything moving. Use this time to get your mind right by going over your workout and what you want to achieve. Find the mind-body connection and concentrate on the things you will achieve that day. This is a great time to visualize your successes and focus on making some great progress.

> *TIP:* Walk to the gym if you can; 1–2 miles of walking will raise your body temperature, engage your core and warm up your legs. Aside from the physical benefits, this is a great way to clear your mind and mentally prepare before a workout and to cool down and loosen up tight muscles on your way home.

"Poor Man's Yoga" Dynamic Warm-Up: Once you've completed the basic warm-up, use the "Poor Man's Yoga" Dynamic Warm-Up on page 149. This sequence of movements will get your lower body ready. This is NOT to be used in place of warm-up sets for squats, deadlifts or other exercises. Rather, this is about making sure the muscles, tendons and ligaments have full range of motion and sufficient pliability for your workout. Remember, this isn't a stretch per se; it's a fluid series of sequential movements to work your body on multiple planes, using multiple muscles across multiple joints—the true definition of a dynamic compound movement.

We like to call this the "Poor Man's Yoga Sequence" because it's a combination of moves that requires balance, flexibility and strength while providing great post–warm up dynamic activation of your lower body and core. Here's the general overview:

In one controlled, sequential movement, you'll stand up straight, bring one knee to chest, release and step into a forward lunge. Then step forward with your opposite foot and stand straight up, bend at the waist and lower your head to knees while keeping your knees straight. Sounds easy, right?

We greatly recommend that you practice all three of these moves by themselves before you do them in combination, especially the lunge. Like any other exercise, performing warm-ups, stretches or dynamic movements like these is a complete waste of time and can potentially cause an injury if done with bad form. Bad lunge form can cause you to bow your upward knee inward and potentially damage your knee—bad news. Plus, you may need to build up your balance from position to position in order to maintain proper form. Take your time, learn how to do it right and then worry about adding intensity or frequency. Don't rush movements simply to move on; just focus on doing them correctly and it will become second nature.

After you've completed the "yoga" sequence, be sure to also warm up your upper body with the movements on pages 151–54.

"Poor Man's Yoga" Dynamic Warm-Up

This sequence will get the muscles and joints of your lower body ready for the workout. Be sure to perform each movement carefully and correctly to maximize the benefits.

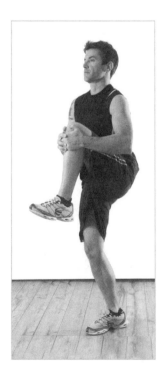

1 Stand up straight in an "athletic stance"; shoulders back, head high, back straight, hands at sides, knees with a slight bend, feet about shoulder-width apart with toes pointed slightly outward. Shift your weight to your right foot while bending your left knee and bringing it up toward your chest. Place your hands on your upper shin, below your knee, and slowly apply force to bring your knee closer to your upper torso while maintaining your balance. Release your left leg if you lose your balance; do not allow your right knee to bow inward or outward as it may result in injury.

2 Slowly, in a controlled manner, release your hands and step forward about 2 feet with your left foot and place it on the ground; drop your hips straight down into a lunge position. Your left leg should be bent 90 degrees, your upper leg parallel with the ground, lower leg perpendicular to it. Your right toes should be on the ground, your right leg bent at 90 degrees as well. Your upper body should be upright, with your head high, shoulders back and core braced to keep your back straight.

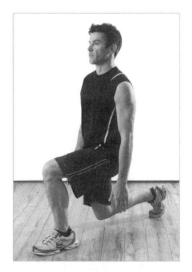

3 Slowly press up from your left heel and push your body back into a standing position with both feet parallel. Bend at the waist and bring your head toward your knees, placing your hands on the backs of your lower calves and pulling slightly to assist in getting your noggin closer to your knees. Release your hands and slowly return to starting position. That's 1 rep; repeat with your right leg. Perform 5 reps on each side.

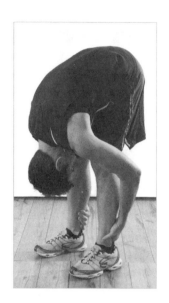

TIP: Never bounce or yank with your arms to pull yourself into position. Perform each move in a slow, controlled, fluid motion. As you repeat, each subsequent movement should provide a little deeper range of motion.

Upper Body Dynamic Warm-Up

Prior to all the lifting and pulling your upper body will do, it's a very good idea to get the muscles loose before beginning the workout. After your basic warm-up period and the yoga-like move (page 149) for the lower body is complete, work through the following movements to prepare your arms, shoulders, chest and back for some serious lifting. The exercises on the next few pages also serve as great stretches for your entire body after you're done with your workout.

Arms across Chest

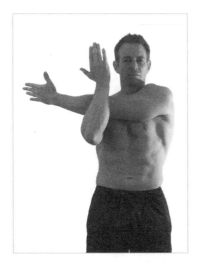 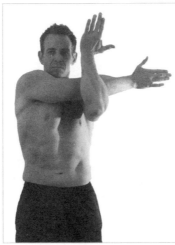

1 Stand with your feet shoulder-width apart and bring your left arm across your chest. Support your left elbow with the crook of your right arm by raising your right arm to 90 degrees. Gently pull your left arm to your chest while maintaining proper posture (straight back, wide shoulders). Don't round or hunch your shoulders. Hold your arm to your chest for 10 seconds.

2 Release and switch arms.

After you've done both sides, shake your hands out for 5–10 seconds.

Chest

1 Clasp your hands together behind your lower back with palms facing each other. Keeping an erect posture and your arms as straight as possible, gently pull your arms away from your back straight out behind you. Keep your shoulders down. Hold for 10 seconds.

Rest for 30 seconds and repeat.

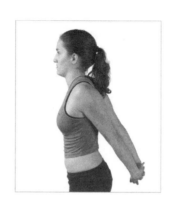

Shoulders & Upper Back

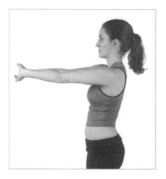
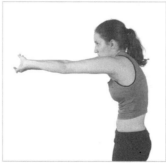

1 Stand with your feet shoulder-width apart and extend both arms straight out in front of you. Interlace your fingers and turn your palms to face away from your body. Keep your back straight.

2 Reach your palms away from your body. Exhale as you push your palms straight out from your body by pushing through your shoulders and upper back. Allow your neck to bend naturally as you round your upper back. Continue to reach your hands and stretch for 10 seconds.

Rest for 30 seconds then repeat. After you've done the second set, shake your arms out to your sides for 10 seconds to return blood to the fingers and forearm muscles.

Arm Circles

1 Stand with your feet shoulder-width apart.

2–3 Move both arms in a complete circle forward 5 times and then backward 5 times

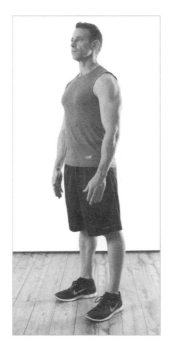
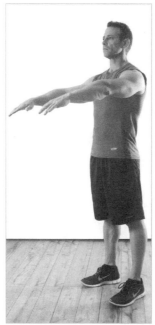
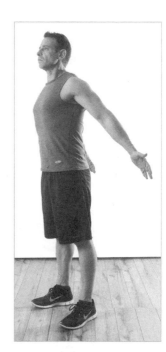

Around the World

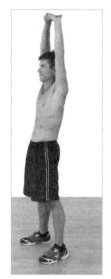

1 Stand with your feet shoulder-width apart and extend your hands overhead with elbows locked, fingers interlocked, and palms up. Keep your arms straight the entire time.

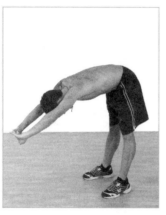

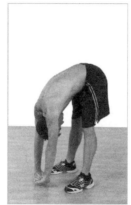

2–3 Bending at the hips, bring your hands down toward your right leg and, in a continuous circular motion, bring your hands toward your toes, then toward your left leg and then return your hands overhead and bend backward.

Repeat three times, then change directions.

Lumber Jack

1 Stand with your feet shoulder-width apart and extend your hands overhead with elbows locked, fingers interlocked, and palms up.

2 Bend forward at the waist and try to put your hands on the ground (like you're chopping wood). Raise up and repeat.

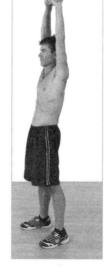

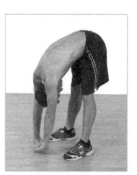

Child's Pose

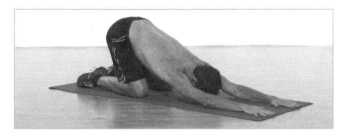

THE POSITION: From a kneeling position, sit your butt back on your calves, then lean forward and place your lower torso on your thighs. Extend your arms directly out in front of you, parallel to each other, and lower your chest toward the floor. Reach your arms as far forward as you can, and rest your forearms and hands flat on the floor. Hold for 30 seconds. Release and then rest for 10 seconds.

Cobra

This stretches and strengthens your abs and back and is a great way to cool down between sets of multiple repetitions.

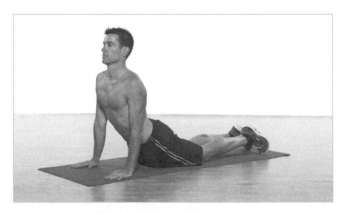

THE POSITION: Lying on your stomach, place your hands directly under your shoulders with your fingers facing forward. Straighten your legs and point your toes. Exhale and engage your core while lifting your chest off the floor and pushing your hips gently into the floor. Your arms help guide you through the movement, and your elbows should remain slightly bent at the top of the extension; your hips should remain in contact with the mat. Hold the "up" position for 15–30 seconds, then gently roll your upper body back to the floor. Rest for 10 seconds.

Index

Photo Credits

Interior photographs are © Scott E. Whitney except as noted below:

page 6: push-up © Nejron Photo/shutterstock.com

page 20: muscle anatomy © photobank.kiev.ua/shutterstock.com

page 38: EZ curl barbell bench press in gym © Mircea Netval/
shutterstock.com

page 64: woman lifting barbell © Ammentorp Photography/
shutterstock.com

page 84: man doing leg press © Alexander Trinitatov/
shutterstock.com

page 100: overhead press with dumbells © mashurov/
shutterstock.com

page 120: woman doing leg press © Minerva Studio/shutterstock
.com

page 121: hamstring curl © Philip Date/shutterstock.com

page 138: © Rapt Productions

page 139: © Rapt Productions

page 144: muscluar man holding weight © cirkoglu/shutterstock
.com

page 152: © Rapt Productions

page 154: © Rapt Productions

page 155: © Rapt Productions

Acknowledgments

A huge thanks to Corey Irwin from both of us. Without your tireless efforts to continually rework the nutrition for this program, we'd have been in a pickle, or in some real hot sauce, but surely in a jam. (Had enough of the food puns?) Sincerely, thank you so much. We're both honored to have you on our tea. Oops, we mean "team."

Brett: To Jason, I still think you're a bit crazy but I'm very grateful that you worked so hard on creating this program and even converting me into a bit more of a weightlifter. I love what it has done for my strength and physique, and I hope everyone who picks up this book gets the same (or better) amazing results! I would also like to thank Mike DeAngelo for introducing me to functional fitness and throwing tons of challenges at me both at the ESPN Health & Fitness Center and at triathlons, duathlons and even our famous Castle Craig double-ascents. MikeyD, you've continued to raise the bar on being an amazing trainer and fitness role model—I'd never be where I am today without your help. To Chris Goggin, Brian Burns and Brooks Warner, you all helped convince me that moving some heavy weights around wasn't such a bad idea. All my love to Kristen, Ian and Vivi for their support.

Jason: To Brooks (my younger brother) and Sloane (my younger sister) for never letting me build an ego. Your continued loving harassment pushed me forward when I wanted to quit! And to my wife Anne-Marie, for putting up with nearly a year of crazy eating, new workout regimes and completely off-the-mark "trial periods." Thanks for the support and not taking the kids and running away!

About the Authors

Brett Stewart is an endurance athlete and certified personal trainer residing in Phoenix, Arizona. An adrenaline junkie, Brett is an Ironman triathlete, ultra-marathoner, and rabid obstacle racer. A proud father, husband, son and brother, Brett has written numerous fitness books including *7 Weeks to a Triathlon*, *7 Weeks to Getting Ripped* and *Ultimate Obstacle Race Training*.

Jason Warner is an ISSA Certified Strength Trainer, fitness and sports enthusiast, ultra-marathoner, triathlete, CrossFitter and overall Olympic-lifting nut. He recently relocated to Victoria, British Columbia, from Adelaide, South Australia, with his wife and two young children. Jason wrote *Ultimate Jump Rope Workouts* and contributed heavily to *7 Weeks to 50 Pull-Ups* and *7 Weeks to Getting Ripped*.

The authors can be contacted online at www.7weekstofitness.com.